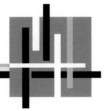

# HANDBOOK OF PSYCHIATRIC EDUCATION

**Second Edition**

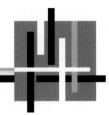

# HANDBOOK OF PSYCHIATRIC EDUCATION

## Second Edition

*Edited by*

Donna M. Sudak, M.D.

AMERICAN PSYCHIATRIC ASSOCIATION PUBLISHING

Second Edition

Manufactured in the United States of America on acid-free paper

25 24 23 22 21 5 4 3 2 1

American Psychiatric Association Publishing
800 Maine Avenue SW, Suite 900
Washington, DC 20024-2812
www.appi.org

**Library of Congress Cataloging-in-Publication Data**

Names: Sudak, Donna M., editor. | American Psychiatric Association, issuing body.
Title: Handbook of psychiatric education / edited by Donna M. Sudak.
Description: Second edition. | Washington, DC : American Psychiatric Association Publishing, [2021] | Includes bibliographical references and index.
Identifiers: LCCN 2020057226 (print) | LCCN 2020057227 (ebook) | ISBN 9781615373444 (paperback ; alk. paper) | ISBN 9781615373826 (ebook)
Subjects: MESH: Psychiatry–education | Education, Medical | United States
Classification: LCC RC459 (print) | LCC RC459 (ebook) | NLM WM 18 | DDC 616.890071–dc23
LC record available at https://lccn.loc.gov/2020057226
LC ebook record available at https://lccn.loc.gov/2020057227

**British Library Cataloguing in Publication Data**

A CIP record is available from the British Library.

# Contents

## Part II

Medical Student Education

## Part III

Resident and Fellowship Education

# CONTRIBUTORS

**Adrienne Adams, M.D., M.S.**
Training Director, Child and Adolescent Psychiatry Fellowship, Department of Psychiatry and Behavioral Sciences, Rush University Medical Center, Chicago, Illinois

**Joan M. Anzia, M.D.**
Professor, Department of Psychiatry and Behavioral Sciences, and Vice Chair for Education, Northwestern University/Feinberg School of Medicine, Chicago, Illinois

**Melissa R. Arbuckle, M.D., Ph.D.**
Vice Chair for Education and Director of Resident Education, Department of Psychiatry, Columbia University Irving Medical Center and the New York State Psychiatric Institute, New York

**Robert N. Averbuch, M.D.**
Associate Professor, Department of Psychiatry, and Associate Residency Training Director, University of Florida College of Medicine, Gainesville, Florida

**Carol A. Bernstein, M.D.**
Professor and Vice Chair, Faculty Development and Wellbeing, Departments of Psychiatry and Behavioral Science and Obstetrics and Gynecology and Women's Health, Montefiore Medical Center/Albert Einstein College of Medicine, Bronx, New York

**Laurel J. Bessey, M.D.**
Clinical Assistant Professor of Psychiatry and Associate Residency Training Director, University of Wisconsin School of Medicine and Public Health, Madison, Wisconsin

**Adam Brenner, M.D.**
Distinguished Teaching Professor, Department of Psychiatry, University of Texas Southwestern Medical Center, Dallas, Texas

**Mary "Molly" Camp, M.D.**
Associate Professor, Department of Psychiatry, University of Texas Southwestern Medical Center, Dallas, Texas

**Kim-Lan Czelusta, M.D.**
Associate Professor and Vice Chair for Education, Menninger Department of Psychiatry and Behavioral Sciences, Baylor College of Medicine, Houston, Texas

**Sandra M. DeJong, M.D., M.Sc.**
Senior Consultant, Child/Adolescent Psychiatry, Cambridge Health Alliance; Assistant Professor, Department of Psychiatry, Harvard Medical School, Cambridge, Massachusetts

**Sallie G. DeGolia, M.D., M.P.H.**
Clinical Professor; Associate Training Director, Adult Psychiatry Program; and Associate Chair for Clinician Educator Faculty Development, Department of Psychiatry and Behavioral Sciences, Stanford University, Stanford, California

**Carrie Ernst, M.D.**
Associate Professor of Psychiatry, Icahn School of Medicine at Mount Sinai, Mount Sinai, New York

**Daniel E. Gih, M.D.**
Associate Professor, Department of Psychiatry, University of Nebraska Medical Center, Omaha, Nebraska

**Sharon Hammer, M.D.**
Assistant Professor, Department of Psychiatry, University of Nebraska Medical Center, Omaha, Nebraska

**John Hearn, M.D.**
Assistant Professor of Psychiatry, Saint Louis University, Saint Louis, Missouri

**Richard C. Holbert, M.D.**
Associate Professor, Department of Psychiatry, University of Florida College of Medicine, Gainesville, Florida

**Jacqueline A. Hobbs, M.D., Ph.D.**
Associate Professor, Vice Chair for Education, and Director, Residency Training Program, Department of Psychiatry, University of Florida College of Medicine, Gainesville, Florida

**Gary L. Kanter, M.D.**
Associate Professor, Department of Psychiatry, University of Florida College of Medicine, Gainesville, Florida

**Anna Kerlek, M.D.**
Assistant Professor of Psychiatry, The Ohio State University, Columbus, Ohio

**Jessica Kovach, M.D.**
Professor of Psychiatry and Behavioral Sciences, Director of Residency Training, and Vice Chairperson, Lewis Katz School of Medicine, Temple University, Philadelphia, Pennsylvania

**Alex Loeks-Johnson, M.D.**
PGY2 Resident, Department of Psychiatry and Behavioral Sciences, University of Minnesota, Minneapolis, Minnesota

**Francis Lu, M.D.**
Luke and Grace Kim Professor in Cultural Psychiatry, Emeritus, University of California, Davis, California

**Vishal Madaan, M.D.**
Associate Professor, Department of Psychiatry and Neurobehavioral Sciences, and Training Director, Child and Adolescent Psychiatry Fellowship, University of Virginia Health System, Charlottesville, Virginia

**Anne McBride, M.D.**
Associate Professor of Psychiatry, University of California, Davis, California

**Katharine J. Nelson, M.D.**
Vice Chair for Education, Department of Psychiatry and Behavioral Sciences; Associate Designated Institutional Official, University of Minnesota Medical School, Minneapolis, Minnesota

**William Newman, M.D.**
Professor of Psychiatry and Interim Chair of Psychiatry, Saint Louis University, Saint Louis, Missouri

**Bianca Baotran T. Nguyen, M.D., M.P.H.**
Postdoctoral Clinical Fellow, Department of Psychiatry, Columbia University Irving Medical Center and the New York State Psychiatric Institute, New York

**John Spollen, M.D.**
Professor and Vice Chair for Education, Department of Psychiatry, College of Medicine, University of Arkansas for Medical Sciences, Little Rock, Arkansas

**Colin Stewart, M.D.**
Training Director, Department of Child and Adolescent Psychiatry; Clerkship Director, Department of Psychiatry; and Associate Professor of Clinical Psychiatry, Georgetown University Medical Center and School of Medicine, Washington, DC

**Sheritta Strong, M.D.**
Assistant Professor, Department of Psychiatry, University of Nebraska Medical Center, Omaha, Nebraska

**Donna M. Sudak, M.D.**
Professor of Psychiatry, Vice Chair for Education and Psychiatry, Drexel University College of Medicine; Program Director, Tower Health–Brandywine Hospital General Psychiatry Residency, Philadelphia, Pennsylvania

**Lia A. Thomas, M.D.**
Medical Director, Mental Health Trauma Services Team, VA North Texas Health Care System–Dallas VA Medical Center; Associate Residency Training Director and Associate Professor, Department of Psychiatry, UT Southwestern Medical Center, Dallas, Texas

**Art Walaszek, M.D.**
Professor of Psychiatry and Residency Training Director, University of Wisconsin School of Medicine and Public Health, Madison, Wisconsin

**Herbert E. Ward Jr., M.D.**
Kaine Professor, Department of Psychiatry, University of Florida College of Medicine, Gainesville, Florida

**Randon S. Welton, M.D.**
Professor and Margaret Clark Morgan Chair of Psychiatry, Northeast Ohio Medical University, Rootstown, Ohio

**Lora Wichser, M.D.**
Deputy Vice Chair for Education, Department of Psychiatry and Behavioral Sciences; Program Director, Psychiatry Residency; Director, Medical Student Psychiatry Clerkship, University of Minnesota Medical School, Minneapolis, Minnesota

# INTRODUCTION

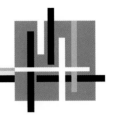

**Psychiatric** education has increased in complexity and content since the previous edition of this book. Much like our learners, educators must contend with a staggering amount of educational content, new teaching methodologies, regulatory requirements, and application inflation. The excitement of engaging new learners is often offset by an overwhelming sense of information overload. My fellow authors and I endeavor to bring some sense of order to this chaos.

The book is divided into three parts. Part I reviews general educational topics. We introduce general scholarship about adult learning principles; navigate the terrain between mentorship, boundaries, and supervision; and share models for a principle-driven approach to educational scholarship. Professionalism and well-being are other key chapters in this section.

Part II covers issues germane to medical student education. These include curricular and clerkship management, special considerations in contemporary undergraduate medical education, evaluation strategies, and the crossover topic of recruiting and advising medical students into psychiatry graduate medical education.

Part III relates to graduate training in psychiatry. Administration, financing and regulatory requirements, curriculum development, specific strategies for managing the problem trainee, and fellowship training are the major topic areas covered. The book concludes with a chapter on career development in psychiatric education.

Each author has made a considerable effort to provide references to Web-based content so that readers may obtain the most current information about training and use the principles in each chapter with the most current regulations and guidelines. We wanted the book to be useful as the landscape changes with time.

Two more points are noteworthy. First, the chapter authors' enthusiasm for educational excellence shines through. We hope to impart this quality to future leaders in psychiatric education. Second, this same passion made the book an utter joy to edit, and I am in the authors' debt.

# PART I

# GENERAL TOPICS IN PSYCHIATRIC EDUCATION

## CHAPTER 1

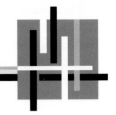

# PRINCIPLES OF ADULT LEARNING

Bianca Baotran T. Nguyen, M.D., M.P.H.
Melissa R. Arbuckle, M.D., Ph.D.

**In** the late Middle Ages, doctors in training primarily acquired knowledge and skills through apprenticeship, a dyadic arrangement of novice learner and master physician for the transfer of information. In the half a millennium since then, medical education has dramatically evolved from textbooks, university lectures, and bedside teaching on academic wards to now instantly available innumerable online resources, videos, and modules. Concurrently, the field of psychiatry is rapidly expanding, with advances in neuroscience and genetics and new models for patient care delivery, such as integrated care and telehealth. Psychiatrists must navigate this ever-changing landscape and determine training priorities, identify resources, efficiently retrieve information, assess outcomes, and assimilate learning into clinical practice. The application of adult learning principles to clinical training in psychiatry is critical to help learners keep pace with this new "information age" and develop the skills necessary for lifelong learning.

## FOUNDATIONS OF ADULT LEARNING

*Andragogy*, which is derived from the Greek *andr-*, meaning "man," and *agogos*, meaning "to lead," was popularized by Malcolm Knowles in the 1980s as a term referring to the principles of adult learning. Based on the premise that adults are intrinsically motivated and self-directed, he established four assumptions about adult learners, adding a fifth later (Knowles 1984):

1. **Self-concept:** Adults are self-directed and take ownership of learning as they grow and develop a sense of self and individual preferences.
2. **Experience:** Adults draw on varying degrees of accumulated knowledge and past experiences to enhance learning.
3. **Readiness to learn:** Adults' circumstances and developmental tasks often change as they progress through new social roles. They value learning knowledge and skills that are most applicable to their current stage of training and responsibilities.
4. **Orientation to learning:** Adults desire immediate and practical application of information. They are problem oriented as opposed to content oriented.
5. **Motivation to learn:** Adults are intrinsically motivated, for example, by purpose, job satisfaction, mastery, and a sense of relatedness or belonging.

These concepts may sound familiar given the inherent use of adult learning principles in our therapeutic work with patients. We deliver well-timed interventions when aligned with a patient's intrinsic motivation, provide supportive interventions that promote autonomy, and adapt our approach based on thoughtful assessment of a patient's individual needs, goals, and circumstances.

Although Knowles's andragogical principles form the foundation for adult learning theory, these tenets lack substantial empirical support and are by no means all-inclusive. Extrinsic motivation, reflection, and sociocultural contexts also have a role in shaping how adults learn. Beyond andragogy, alternative theories of adult and general learning theory abound. Behaviorist theories of learning suggest that behavioral change is shaped by classical and operant conditioning (Mann 2004). Cognitive theories focus on the extent to which cognitive processes (e.g., registering, understanding, retaining, and recalling information) influence learning. Constructivism, a cognitive theory of learning described by Jean Piaget, suggests that learners process new information through pre-formed cognitive assumptions developed from past experiences (Powell et al. 2009). Relational theories, such as situated cognition, consider learning to be a social activity dependent on individualized context and environment (Brown et al. 1989). Other theories include transformative learning theory, a model that leverages critical reflection to change one's perspective and worldview, and self-determination theory, which emphasizes the connection between motivation and expectation of learning in driving the pursuit of knowledge (Taylor and Hamdy 2013).

In the sections that follow, we link theory to practice and offer suggestions for incorporating adult learning principles into psychiatric education. Just as a firm grasp of psychotherapy theory grounds practice and guides effective treatment, application of adult learning theory can improve educational interventions. Adult learning principles can inform approaches to teaching and enrich teaching methods used in the classroom or clinical setting.

## APPLYING ADULT LEARNING PRINCIPLES AT THE LEVEL OF EDUCATOR AND TRAINEE

In a review of 68 articles exploring what factors make "a good clinical teacher in medicine," the five most commonly reported themes (Sutkin et al. 2008) were

1. Medical/clinical knowledge
2. Clinical and technical skills/competence and clinical reasoning
3. Positive relationships with students and a supportive learning environment
4. Communication skills
5. Enthusiasm

Not surprisingly, a natural connection occurs between what adults want from their teachers and adult learning theory. Proficient, competent educators model achievement and inspire attainment of excellence, motivating trainees to set increasingly higher goals. Enthusiastic and effective communicators expertly appeal to their trainees' needs, show why material is relevant, and foster trainees' personal connection to the subject matter by drawing on their personal experiences and prior knowledge. Using Knowles's (1984) assumptions about adult learners, Table 1–1 lists implications for goals in teaching and practical applications for psychiatric education.

**Table 1–1.** Applying Knowles's andragogical principles to psychiatric education

| Goals in teaching | Clinical educating methods |
|---|---|
| **Self-concept:** Encourage individual inquiry and self-directed learning | Ask trainees to state their own goals and priorities for learning at the start of a class/rotation or before initiating a patient interview |
| | Use a graduated approach, offering more clinical responsibility and less direct supervision over time |
| | Challenge trainees to make decisions (e.g., regarding diagnosis or treatment choices) and discuss their rationale |
| | Ask for trainees' input and opinions often |
| | Provide useful resources early on that trainees can access independently on their own time |
| **Experience:** Acknowledge and validate learners' individual backgrounds, experiences, and prior knowledge | Create a cooperative learning environment built on mutual respect |
| | Share past learning experiences as appropriate, and invite trainees to share their own as it relates to learning |
| | Facilitate reflection: ask trainees to compare prior experiences and knowledge to what they are learning |
| | Link learning material to trainees' interests |
| | Universalize the concept that individuals hold implicit biases, and model ways to bring bias into awareness and to mitigate its impact on patient care |
| | Reassure trainees that there are many different approaches to subjective aspects of clinical practice and not necessarily any one *right* way of doing things |
| **Readiness to learn:** Modify educational materials and content based on the learner's level of training | Assess trainees' needs |
| | List learning objectives at the start of every learning experience, whether it occurs more formally in a classroom or on bedside rounds |
| | Gauge receptiveness to learning by attending to trainees' affect and cognitive-emotional state |

**Table 1–1.** Applying Knowles's andragogical principles to psychiatric education *(continued)*

| Goals in teaching | Clinical educating methods |
|---|---|
| **Readiness to learn** *(continued)* | Consider how much time trainees can dedicate to self-study and adapt teaching methods accordingly (i.e., residents often lack time for class preparation given clinical duties compared with preclinical medical students) |
| **Orientation to learning:** Prioritize relevant, practical, and problem-centered material that can be immediately applicable to real clinical scenarios | Start instruction by posing a problem and providing educational material for learners to solve it |
| | Provide or ask trainees to contribute personal examples and case studies that demonstrate practical application of theories and techniques |
| | Leverage unexpected "teachable moments" to deepen learning relevant to a distinct time, place, and situation |
| | Keep teaching points brief, succinct, and time limited |
| | Engage multidisciplinary staff in teaching trainees during their interactions (e.g., have social workers review disposition planning or nurses explain the floor protocol for admissions) |
| **Motivation to learn:** Guide trainees in achieving competence while bolstering their intrinsic motivation and supporting self-esteem | Give specific and objective feedback that highlights strengths and offers suggestions for improvement |
| | Link learning objectives to trainees' long-term plans and expectations |
| | Provide methods for self-assessment |
| | Stimulate interest by demonstrating genuine enthusiasm and excitement |
| | Diversify teaching methods (e.g., online applications, pair-sharing, writing exercises) and allow trainees' flexibility in choice with regard to how they want to learn |

## APPLYING ADULT LEARNING PRINCIPLES ACROSS VARIOUS SETTINGS

Adult learning principles support the notion that the process of achieving professional competence is adaptive and developmental and may be integrated into multiple teaching formats, including classroom, clinical setting, and self-study.

### Classroom

A traditional classroom implies a formal frame, with a predetermined setting and topic and teacher-led learning. To embody adult learning principles, classroom teaching should engage the student as much as possible in the process of active learning.

#### *LECTURES*

The lights dim, a slide is enlarged on the screen, and a familiar yellow, serif font appears across a dark blue background. Stereotypically, lectures feature passive learners who face the educator and a static screen. Lectures are still the predominant method of teaching from preclinical years through residents' didactic curriculum and have the advantages of disseminating knowledge from one to many, introducing or deepening learning on complex and difficult topics, and conveying the instructor's personal perspective (Palis and Quiros 2014). However, lectures can and should employ adult learning principles to facilitate active learning. Engaging trainees in the interpretation and assessment of lecture content may potentially improve the knowledge retention rate, which is estimated at a disheartening 5% after traditional lectures (Masters 2013). Cooper and Richards (2017) outlined several active learning strategies that can be incorporated to improve lectures:

1. *Break long lectures into shorter segments with paired or group activities.* The average adult learner's attention span is estimated at 10–15 minutes (Jeffries 2014). Limits of working memory and decreased ability to meaningfully assimilate new information (also known as *interference*) detrimentally impact attention and retention. Implement think-pair-share activities every 15 minutes. These activities ask learners to *think* about content learned and questions raised, discuss and compare these concepts in *pairs*, and *share* their consensus with the entire group.
2. *Elicit responses from the audience.* Pose questions to listeners throughout the lecture using technological platforms (e.g., online polls or "click-

ers"), paper, or a show of hands. Responses obtained with a preassessment offer the opportunity to tailor the material to trainee needs. Assess past experience as well; ask if trainees have encountered similar problems before and how they handled them. For example, during a lecture on the management of alcohol withdrawal, residents may have experience using chlordiazepoxide but have not yet treated alcohol withdrawal with intravenous benzodiazepines. A trainee who is asked and is unsure about benzodiazepine equivalents conversions may review and bookmark resources for later reference. Questions asked during and after the lecture stimulate interest, self-assessment, and motivation to reinforce learning lecture content.

3. *Be ACTIVE.* A group of residents and faculty developed ACTIVE, a structured lecture format that incorporates principles of adult learning. Trainees **A**ssemble into small groups. The educator **C**onveys three to five learning points and **T**eaches a limited amount of content. The educator then **I**nquires about how the material applies to a clinical scenario, **V**erifies learning after discussion of each group's answers, and **E**xplains and educates how the answer choices reflect the learning points (Sawatsky et al. 2014). Discussion of a clinical scenario makes learning problem centered rather than content centered, which is appealing to adults who require immediacy of application.

## *FLIPPED CLASSROOM*

Traditionally, trainees learn from teachers in a classroom and bring materials home to study and review. In a flipped classroom model, trainees learn material on their own and build on what they learned in the classroom through individual exploration or group activities. For example, rather than learning about prescribing practices for antidepressants in a lecture, residents might complete a preclass worksheet focused on the indications, adverse effects, and dosage recommendations of the antidepressants. Residents then come to class, break into small groups, and roleplay as prescribers and patients who are initiating treatment for depression (Kavanagh et al. 2017).

Teachers who use a flipped classroom approach facilitate learning rather than directly instructing, encouraging trainees to move at their own pace. A meta-analysis published in 2018 found that students favor a flipped classroom over a traditional classroom and that the flipped classroom model was more effective in increasing student learning (Hew and Lo 2018). Residents and medical students have little free time to study outside of rotations, especially for topics that do not pertain to their immediate clinical needs. Thus, the flipped classroom model may be modified to include a "prelearning" period during allotted class time rather than outside of class. Alternatively, preclass material such as video clips, podcasts, or Web-based modules should be limited (lasting no longer than 10–15 minutes), and learners should be given an estimate of how long this preparatory work will take. Done well, a flipped classroom approach may accelerate mastery through imminent transfer to practice and bolster intrinsic motivation as trainees progress toward competency (Persky and McLaughlin 2017).

### *SIMULATION AND STANDARDIZED PATIENTS*

Residents' clinical experience is tied to the presentation and pathology of their assigned patients. Given the 250 psychiatric disorders listed in DSM-5 (American Psychiatric Association 2013) and the myriad available treatments, it is impossible to cover the breadth of psychiatric diagnosis and treatment solely through direct clinical practice. *Simulations*, defined as "approximations to reality that require trainees to react to problems or conditions as they would under genuine circumstances" can fill this gap (Tekian et al. 1999). Simulations broaden exposure to clinical material and provide opportunities for immediate feedback and reflection that are not possible in every patient encounter (Abdool et al. 2017). Experiences with standardized patients may shift trainees' perspectives on bias, stigma, and capacity for empathy. In a safe, trusting, and collaborative simulation environment, transformative learning is promoted through trial and error and reflection (Clapper 2010).

## Clinical Settings

As trainees transition from the classroom to clinical practice, learning shifts from theoretical knowledge to clinical reasoning and practical application. Miller's pyramid (Miller 1990) may guide planning and assessment of clinical competence. In clinical training, students build from a base of knowledge ("knows") and applied knowledge ("knows how") to a demonstration of skills ("shows how") before reaching the apex at which their knowledge and skills are consolidated into clinical practice ("does"). The clinical setting lends itself to informal teaching and numerous opportunities to apply adult learning principles. We focus on bedside teaching and clinical rounds in the following section; supervision is discussed later in Chapter 4.

### *BEDSIDE TEACHING*

The traditional model of apprenticeship—"see one, do one, teach one"—carries into modern-day medical education. Given the affective, subjective, and personalized aspects of psychiatric care, skills are not transferable by passive observation. Active engagement before, during, and after patient interaction is required. Lokko et al. (2016) underscored the importance of keeping bedside teaching "both learner centered and patient centered" and provided a comprehensive overview of how adult learning principles can be incorporated into psychiatric "pre-bedside encounters, bedside encounters, and post-bedside encounters":

1. **Before seeing the patient:** Engage your trainees by asking them to set learning objectives before meeting the patient; refine as necessary. Define a time frame and specific expectations for the interaction. Assign active roles to each participant, depending on level of training and learning goals. For example, the medical student interviews the patient, and a resident observer develops a biopsychosocial formulation.
2. **During the patient encounter:** Capitalize on "teachable moments." Demonstrate an examination skill or ask trainees to do so, model parts of the interview as appropriate, offer affirmation in real time, and give gentle redirection.
3. **After seeing the patient:** Debrief the patient encounter away from the bedside. Encourage reflection and a discussion of "sensitive or affectively charged aspects of the encounter." Explore transference and countertransference to promote transformative learning. Give specific feedback and ask for trainees' feedback on what and how they learned during the patient interaction. Deliver teaching points succinctly and leave trainees with a clinical pearl that they can apply in the future.

### *CLINICAL ROUNDS*

During clinical rounds, trainees may synthesize information by presenting cases and demonstrate competence by sharing input and rationale on diagnostic impressions and treatment decisions. To employ adult learning principles, consider rounds from the learner's perspective with regard to environment, learning objectives, and educational methods. Does the environment feel safe and welcoming of diverse opinions? Invite trainees to sit at the table when presenting a case, to bolster their self-confidence. Ask for their input when staff ask how to respond to a clinical situation. Are trainees' needs and learning goals known? Ask what questions came up during their assessment or presentation. Socratic questioning may identify the extent of trainee knowledge but must be used with care; learners are often frustrated by Socratic questioning that appears as "guess what I'm thinking," and it often implies a performative aspect with a risk of humiliation. Deliver teaching points effectively and timely, with context. Demonstrate respect by acknowledging time constraints and trainees' clinical duties. If rounds end before questions can be discussed, set a convenient time to reconvene.

### Self-Study

In line with the adult learning principle of self-direction, learning is increasingly taking place outside of the classroom. According to a report by the Association of American Medical Colleges (2018) that surveyed second-year students, nearly one-quarter of subjects reported "almost never" attending in-person preclerkship courses or lectures, and the majority (42.4%) reported attending virtual pre-clerkship courses and lectures "most of the time." Educators teaching preclinical courses should consider providing multimedia materials to offer students a choice in learning, for example, lecture slides with audio to teach the mental status examination, along with a video clip of a psychiatrist conducting the examination and related reading materials.

Trainees and practicing psychiatrists must independently determine when acquisition of facts is most useful versus a deeper exploration of concepts, given the overwhelming amount of available content. Studies suggest that problem-based learning can facilitate self-study; trainees are presented with an open-ended problem and subsequently set their own learning objectives and pursue an answer via self-directed learning or group discussion (Wood 2003). Residents who are exposed to problem-based learning dedicate more hours to independent study, have more discussions with co-residents outside of scheduled classes and rounds, and perform more computer literature searches each week (Ozuah et al. 2001). Teaching through problem-based learning models being faced with a clinical problem that requires selection of research materials, independent investigation, and assimilation of knowledge, which furthers lifelong learning.

## CONCLUSION

A practical understanding of adult learning principles lays the groundwork for psychiatric education and facilitates one's development as a clinical educator. Teaching that takes an adaptive, learner-centered, and problem-oriented approach promotes trainees' advancement in self-directed learning, evoking meaning and purpose. Their growth and accomplishment makes teaching generative and immensely rewarding.

## — KEY POINTS —

- Adult learners are self-directed, problem oriented, and intrinsically motivated.
- Trainees use past experiences and knowledge to enhance learning and value relevant, immediate, and practical application of skills and concepts.
- General learning theories, such as humanistic, cognitive, behavioral, and relational models, may be used to understand how trainees learn and to adapt teaching methods accordingly.
- Active learning strategies improve students' engagement in traditional models of teaching, such as lectures and bedside rounds.
- Self-study promotes independent inquiry and lifelong learning skills required by the rapidly evolving advances in psychiatric research and knowledge.

# REFERENCES

Abdool PS, Nirula L, Bonato S, et al: Simulation in undergraduate psychiatry: exploring the depth of learner engagement. Acad Psychiatry 41(2):251–261, 2017

American Psychiatric Association: Diagnostic and Statistical Manual of Mental Disorders, 5th Edition. Arlington, VA, American Psychiatric Association, 2013

Association of American Medical Colleges: Medical School Year Two Questionnaire: 2017 All Schools Summary Report. Washington, DC, Association of American Medical Colleges, 2018. Available at: https://www.aamc.org/system/files/reports/1/y2q2017report.pdf. Accessed August 25, 2019.

Brown JS, Collins A, Duguid P: Situated cognition and the culture of learning. Educ Res 18(1):32–42, 1989

Clapper TC: Beyond Knowles: what those conducting simulation need to know about adult learning theory. Clin Simul Nurs 6(1):e7–e14, 2010

Cooper AZ, Richards JB: Lectures for adult learners: breaking old habits in graduate medical education. Am J Med 130(3):376–381, 2017

Hew KF, Lo CK: Flipped classroom improves student learning in health professions education: a meta-analysis. BMC Med Educ 18(1):38, 2018

Jeffries WB: Teaching large groups, in An Introduction to Medical Teaching. Edited by Huggett KN, Jeffries WB. New York, Springer, 2014, pp 11–26

Kavanagh EP, Cahill J, Arbuckle MR, et al: Psychopharmacology prescribing workshops: a novel method for teaching psychiatry residents how to talk to patients about medications. Acad Psychiatry 41(4):491–496, 2017

Knowles M: The Adult Learner: A Neglected Species. Houston, TX, Gulf Publishing, 1984

Lokko HN, Gatchel JR, Becker MA, Stern TA: The art and science of learning, teaching, and delivering feedback in psychosomatic medicine. Psychosomatics 57(1):31–40, 2016

Mann KV: The role of educational theory in continuing medical education: has it helped us? J Contin Educ Health Prof 24(suppl 1):S22–S30, 2004

Masters K: Edgar Dale's Pyramid of Learning in medical education: a literature review. Med Teach 35(11):e1584–e1593, 2013

Miller GE: The assessment of clinical skills/competence/performance. Acad Med 65(9 suppl):S63–S67, 1990

Ozuah PO, Curtis J, Stein REK: Impact of problem-based learning on residents' self-directed learning. Arch Pediatr Adolesc Med 155(6):669–672, 2001

Palis AG, Quiros PA: Adult learning principles and presentation pearls. Middle East Afr J Ophthalmol 21(2):114–122, 2014

Persky AM, McLaughlin JE: The flipped classroom: from theory to practice in health professional education. Am J Pharm Educ 81(6):118, 2017

Powell KC, Cody ED, Kalina J: Cognitive and social constructivism: developing tools for an effective classroom. Education 130(2):241–250, 2009

Sawatsky AP, Berlacher K, Granieri R: Using an ACTIVE teaching format versus a standard lecture format for increasing resident interaction and knowledge achievement during noon conference: a prospective, controlled study. BMC Med Educ 14:129, 2014

Sutkin G, Wagner E, Harris I, Schiffer R: What makes a good clinical teacher in medicine? A review of the literature. Acad Med 83(5):452–466, 2008

Taylor DCM, Hamdy H: Adult learning theories: implications for learning and teaching in medical education: AMEE Guide No. 83. Med Teach 35(11):e1561–e1572, 2013

Tekian A, McGuire CH, McGaghie WC: Innovative Simulations for Assessing Professional Competence. Chicago, IL, University of Illinois Department of Medical Education, 1999

Wood DF: ABC of learning and teaching in medicine: problem based learning. BMJ 326(7384):328–330, 2003

# CHAPTER 2

# PROFESSIONALISM

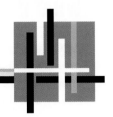

Sandra M. DeJong, M.D., M.Sc.

**Professionalism** is increasingly viewed as core to medical education. However, defining, operationalizing, teaching, and assessing professionalism remain challenging. Professionalism norms and perceptions vary by developmental stage, gender, age, and generation as well as geographical, ethnic, and institutional cultures (Jain et al. 2010; Paauw et al. 2017; Swick 2007). As health care professionals develop over the course of their careers, their views of professionalism may shift (Nath et al. 2006; Wagner et al. 2007). The rise in emphasis on professionalism lies in its potential to address perceived threats in medicine—loss of professional identity, decline in quality, commercialization, technology and loss of humanism—and to prevent future disciplinary actions (Birden et al. 2014; Cruess et al. 2006; Irvine 1999; Papadakis et al. 2005; Relman 2007; Rothman 2000; Swick 2007; Woodruff et al. 2008).

The American Board of Internal Medicine initiated "Project Professionalism" in the 1990s. Guidelines for both undergraduate and graduate medical education thereafter required professionalism education; professionalism became one of the six core competencies across medical specialties introduced by the Accreditation Council for Graduate Medical Education (ACGME) in 1999 and a domain to be evaluated in 2009 (Accreditation Council for Graduate Medical Education 1999; Accreditation Council for Graduate Medical Education and American Board of Psychiatry and Neurology 2015; Rider 2007). Psychiatric residents have expressed the need for professionalism training (Jain et al. 2011).

# WHAT IS PROFESSIONALISM?

A 2014 systematic review and qualitative meta-synthesis of the medical professionalism literature that set out to establish an optimal definition concluded, "The semantics of professionalism obfuscate more than they clarify, and the continually shifting nature of the medical profession and the organizational and social milieu in which it operates creates a dynamic situation where no definition has yet taken hold as the definitive one" (Birden et al. 2014, p. 58). The focus here is on some key conceptual approaches that have emerged in attempting to define professionalism (Table 2–1).

Irby and Hamstra (2016) attempted to organize the professionalism literature into three frameworks: 1) virtue-based professionalism, 2) behavior-based professionalism, and 3) professional identity formation. The virtue-based approach focuses on physicians as people of moral character who, through reasoning and application of ethical principles, act in their patients' best interest over their own. The behavior-based approach, the model adopted by ACGME and other accrediting organizations, focuses on measurable behaviors, milestones, and competencies. Appropriate behavior results from giving clear expectations, feedback on performance, and reinforcement (Accreditation Council for Graduate Medical Education 1999; Accreditation Council for Graduate Medical Education and American Board of Psychiatry and Neurology 2015). The professional identity formation approach combines psychological concepts of identity formation with social learning theory and espouses the unique development of each individual from lay person to physician in the context of a "community of practice" wherein a socialization process utilizing role modeling, direct instruction, coaching, assessment, and feedback occurs (Cruess et al. 2015). These different approaches to defining professionalism overlap in both theory and practice.

In psychiatric education, the explicit teaching about professionalism is often contextual. Early in residency, trainees on intensive services learn about involuntary commitment, confidentiality and when it can be breached, managing risk, and substituted judgment. Training about informed consent in prescribing medications occurs in inpatient and outpatient settings. As they learn psychotherapy, residents begin to appreciate boundary crossings and violations, complex countertransference and its potential enactments, and the importance of maintaining a frame. By doing academic and research projects and participating in journal clubs, residents come to understand research ethics, conflicts of interest, and academic integrity.

**Table 2–1.** Examples of approaches to defining professionalism

| Source | Approach | Explanation (Examples) |
|---|---|---|
| DeJong 2014; Kao 2005 | Compliance with ethical, legal, and professionalism principles | Behavior meets accepted ethical, legal, and professionalism standards as defined by organizational codes of ethics, state medical boards, the law, insurers, and health care institutions (nonmaleficence, confidentiality laws, bans on sexual relationships with patients) |
| International Ottawa Conference Working Group on the Assessment of Professionalism (Hodges et al. 2011) | Individual | Traits, states, behaviors, and cognitive processes of psychiatrists (compassion, integrity, empathic listening, keeping apprised of scientific evidence) |
| | Interpersonal | Psychiatrist–patient, psychiatrist–colleague, and supervisor–trainee relationships (respect for boundaries and power differentials) |
| | Societal-institutional | Relationship with society (advocacy for just distribution of resources; Physicians' Charter, American Board of Internal Medicine Foundation et al. 2002) |
| Irby and Hamstra 2016 | Virtue based | Moral values and reasoning and ethical principles are internalized, resulting in appropriate action (altruism, respect for persons) |
| | Behavior based | Defined competencies and behaviors measure appropriateness of actions ("Performs tasks and responsibilities in a timely manner," PROF 2, Accreditation Council for Graduate Medical Education [2020] milestones, Entrustable Professional Activities [Ten Cate 2006]) |
| | Professional identity formation (Cruess et al. 2015) | Process of individual development from lay person to psychiatrist through socialization in a community of practice with positive role models results in appropriate action |

The principles of professionalism largely transcend differences between medical specialties, as evidenced by the recent "harmonizing" of the milestones under ACGME's professionalism competency across specialties; however, the nature of psychiatric practice and the psychiatrist–patient relationship may necessitate a higher standard of professionalism for psychiatrists (Edgar et al. 2018; Gabbard et al. 2012).

## TEACHING, ASSESSING, AND REMEDIATING PROFESSIONALISM

How to teach professionalism varies with the definition being used. A systematic review of the best evidence for how to teach professionalism identified no gold standard (Birden et al. 2013), but the authors concluded that role modeling and personal reflection under faculty guidance are broadly considered most effective. Experts suggest integrating professionalism throughout the curriculum. Quantitative studies support the following teaching methodologies:

- Faculty–trainee interviews as follow-up to a critical incident report (Baernstein and Fryer-Edwards 2003)
- Vignettes with professionalism dilemmas (although this finding was not generalizable to future scenarios) (Boenink et al. 2005)
- Role modeling, case conferences, and discussions with multidisciplinary experts (in contrast to lectures, videos, and grand rounds) (Roberts et al. 2004)

Observed structured clinical encounters build on case-based teaching and simulation by providing a platform for developing peer feedback skills (Tucker et al. 2017). Qualitative studies identified critical reflection, role modeling, and early clinical experiences as the best teaching methods (Birden et al. 2013).

Proponents of the professional identity formation model advocate for *situated learning theory*, in which teaching is tailored to the institutional environment; is practical, not theoretical; incorporates critical reflection; and follows a "cognitive apprenticeship" model (Cruess et al. 2016b). They also support experiential learning and reflection through the use of art and literature, narrative-based learning, learning portfolios, lectures, panel discussions, small-group courses on reflective medical practice, essays, and whole-class reflection and simulation (see Chapters 5–7). Professionalism-oriented curricula and programs in psychiatry have also been published (Dingle et al. 2016; Lewis and Allan 2016; Moss et al.

2008; Soklaridis et al. 2015). See Table 2–2 for a list of recommended methods.

Assessing professionalism is vital to reassure stakeholders, offer formative guidance and feedback to learners, and place benchmarks in professionalism development for educational planning and certification. Medical schools and residencies now incorporate professionalism assessments into the admissions process; best practices are currently being studied (Schnapp et al. 2019).

How professionalism is defined will determine how it should be assessed. In general, the literature suggests that professionalism may be best evaluated by multiple informants in multiple contexts over time through rigorous analysis and interpretation of data that is systematically collected and results in appropriate interventions. Assessments must be clearly defined as supportive, regulatory, or both and should take place in a safe, nurturing learning environment that also includes faculty development on professionalism. Cultural and generational differences must also be considered (Hodges et al. 2011).

Miller's pyramid, an educationally oriented, oft-cited approach to assessment, takes learners from "knows" through "knows how," "shows how," and "does" (Miller 1990; Norcini and Shea 2016). Cruess et al. (2016a) suggested a fifth level, "is," reflecting the professional identity formation concept. Reliable and valid instruments measuring each of these levels are needed. A systematic review of the quality and utility of observer-based instruments for medical professionals identified 10 instruments (Kwan et al. 2018). The Education Outcomes Services Group Questionnaire and the Professionalism Mini-Evaluation Exercise had the best psychometric properties, and the latter scored higher on utility (Cruess et al. 2006; Kwan et al. 2018). Psychiatric residents may prefer clinical supervision and direct observation for assessment of professionalism (Marrero et al. 2013). For a programmatic assessment approach in psychiatry, see Schuwirth et al. (2017); for a review, see Plakiotis (2017). Table 2–3 provides a list of sample instruments for assessing professionalism.

Professionalism deficits are among the most challenging to remediate, and professionalism is one of the most common reasons for termination from training (Regan et al. 2016). Best practices with a strong evidence base are lacking. Obstacles to remediation include uncertainty about how to define professionalism, a belief that such deficits cannot be fixed, avoidance of confrontation, and a lack of familiarity with procedures and remediation tools.

How one conceptualizes a professionalism lapse may determine the best response. For example, individual factors might result in referring the trainee for neuropsychological testing or psychotherapy or assigning

**Table 2–2.** Teaching methods for psychiatric professionalism

| |
|---|
| **Clinical** |
| Role modeling |
| Supervision that includes a professionalism perspective |
| Faculty–trainee discussion after a critical incident report |
| Observed structured clinical encounters |
| **Didactic** |
| Readings |
| Lectures |
| Large- or small-group discussion using |
| Case conferences |
| Panel discussions with multidisciplinary experts |
| Vignettes with professionalism dilemmas |
| Reflective writing in response to art and literature or other prompts |
| Appreciative inquiry to explore existing practices |
| Roleplay |
| Learning portfolios |
| Essays on topics related to professionalism |
| Whole-class simulation and reflection |

a role model or mentor. One might address a problem in the learning environment via a root cause analysis that leads to systems changes, education, faculty development, or creation of a specific guideline. Response to a problematic interaction might involve team-building exercises or new policies (Arnold et al. 2016). Rougas et al. (2015) offered 12 tips for managing professionalism lapses, and Regan et al. (2016) listed specific remediation strategies. Lapses must be distinguished from stigmatizing personal failures, but communities of practice must establish their own "red line" so that "individuals understand that some kinds of behavior are unacceptable and will not be tolerated" (Arnold et al. 2016, p. 173).

## FACULTY DEVELOPMENT AND THE CLINICAL LEARNING ENVIRONMENT

The clinical learning environment and faculty are integral parts of the teaching and assessment of professionalism (Humphrey et al. 2017; Nordquista et al. 2019; Steinert 2016). On an individual level, faculty development can increase the knowledge, skills, and attitudes required to teach this core competency. In a system, faculty development may artic-

**Table 2–3.** Sample instruments for assessing professionalism

| Instrument (Source) | Format | Additional comments |
|---|---|---|
| Barry Challenges to Professionalism Questionnaire (Barry et al. 2000) | Six patient-based multiple-choice questions, some chosen from American Board of Internal Medicine's Project Professionalism | Brief assessment of professionalism knowledge |
| Conscientiousness Index (McLachlan et al. 2009) | Assessment of key student behaviors, such as attendance at sessions, compliance with paperwork requirements (e.g., immunizations) | Evidence that measures predict professional behavior |
| Critical Incident Technique (Rademacher et al. 2010) | Critical incident brief summary and reflection; analysis and group discussion | Knowledge assessment |
| Jefferson scales (Hojat et al. 2001) | Series of questions with rating scales used to assess empathy, teamwork, and lifelong learning | Strong psychometrics |
| Professionalism-Mini Clinical Evaluation Exercise (Cruess et al. 2006) | Rating of observed behaviors following a brief clinical encounter; feedback and plan for improvement | Evidence of construct and content validity and reasonable interrater reliability; replicated across cultures |
| Situational Judgment Test (McDaniel et al. 2007) | Video recorded or written hypothetical scenarios with responses to be ranked | Strong predictor of work-related outcomes; used in medical school and residency application process |
| Standardized patients (Van Zanten et al. 2005) | Actor-patient clinical encounters scored according to defined professionalism competencies | Validated measure |
| Test of Residents' Ethics Knowledge for Pediatrics (Kesselheim et al. 2012) | 23-Item test on ethics knowledge | Knowledge assessment; potential model for psychiatry |
| 360-Degree evaluations | Collated multisource feedback on professionalism criteria from peers, colleagues, and patients | Improved validity and reliability with increased range of sources |

*Source.* Norcini and Shea 2016.

ulate the organization's desired culture of professionalism and identify factors that enhance or impede its development. Examples of faculty development workshops in psychiatry are available in the literature (e.g., Bursch et al. 2016).

The Liaison Committee on Medical Education (2020) requires that medical schools' learning environments be "conducive to the ongoing development of explicit and appropriate professional behaviors in its medical students, faculty, and staff at all locations" (Standard 3, Element 5, p. 4). The Association of American Medical Colleges (2018) issues an annual report of graduates' experience of the learning environment, including professionalism. The ACGME identifies professionalism as one of the six focus areas for the Clinical Learning Environment Review program (Weiss et al. 2013). Nonetheless, reviews of these environments elicit reports of disruptive or disrespectful behavior on the part of clinical staff. Residents and fellows report having to compromise their integrity to satisfy an authority figure. Most clinical learning environments lack a shared understanding for resolving perceived mistreatment (Bagian and Weiss 2016; Mavis et al. 2014).

When asked about professionalism, learners often cite inconsistencies between what they are taught and what they experience. This discrepancy represents the "hidden curriculum," the "cultural mores that are transmitted but not openly acknowledged through the formal and informal curriculum" (Hafferty and Hafler 2011, p. 17). This "do as I say, not as I do" culture frustrates new learners, who report that such experiences can negate the compassion they felt when they entered the field and undercut explicit professionalism teaching (Gupta et al. 2016; Stephenson et al. 2006; Wear et al. 2008). Gabbard et al. (2012) described ethical tensions inherent in the hidden curriculum of psychiatry training.

Systems issues in the learning environment may limit the capacity of learners to demonstrate professionalism and to report systems problems and faculty professionalism lapses (Hodges et al. 2016). Instruments to assess the extent to which clinical learning environments support reporting concerns about unprofessional behavior are being developed (Martinez et al. 2015).

## PROFESSIONALISM TOPICS IN PSYCHIATRY FOR THE TWENTY-FIRST CENTURY

Certain topics have risen in importance in thinking about professionalism education in psychiatry. These include digital technology and "e-professionalism"; diversity, equity, and inclusion; and interprofessional collaboration. As the digital revolution has rapidly advanced, so too have digital professionalism concerns: online professionalism lapses (Chretien et al. 2009; Greysen et al. 2012); challenges to standards such as privacy and boundaries (Gabbard 2019; Gabbard et al. 2012); inconsistent evidence for online and application-based treatments (Bakker et al. 2016; Larsen et al. 2019); cybersecurity (Huckvale et al. 2019); and professional standards for providing e-behavioral health care and curating an online identity (Hilty et al. 2015, 2019; Liu et al. 2019; Maheu et al. 2018). Professionalism training must include these topics; competencies are being defined and educational resources developed (DeJong 2014; DeJong et al. 2012).

Along with changing demographics, culture, diversity, equity and inclusion, and structural competence are also now key elements of professionalism. The practice of psychiatry inherently involves developing an intimate understanding of those who are different from ourselves (Gabbard et al. 2012). Awareness of health care disparities, including in mental health, has grown (Institute of Medicine Committee on Understanding and Eliminating Racial and Ethnic Disparities in Health Care 2003). Understanding these and advocating for social justice are current tenets of professionalism and professionalism education (Bromage et al. 2019; Higginbotham 2017). Implicit bias includes stigma against mental illness, which also occurs among mental health professionals and may impede psychiatrists from accessing help for their own personal mental health concerns (McLeary-Gaddy et al. 2019).

Finally, learning to work in multidisciplinary teams, long integral to psychiatry training and clinical practice, is more pressing given current workforce shortages and the advent of integrated and collaborative care, accountable care organizations, and other health care delivery systems. The Interprofessional Education Collaborative (2011) defined *interprofessional professionalism* and its core competencies. Professionalism experts describe professional identity formation in this interprofessional context (Hammick et al. 2009; Molleman and Rink 2013; Thistlethwaite et al. 2016). Continuing efforts to define, teach, and assess professionalism in the context of an ever-changing learning environment will undoubtedly serve as "drivers of change" in this critical area of psychiatry (Birden et al. 2014).

## —KEY POINTS—

- No consensus exists for defining professionalism in medical education; various models of professionalism emphasize different domains.

- Proposed frameworks of professionalism include the virtue-based, behavior-based, and professional identity formation approaches; the latter is a developmental model that emphasizes the role of environmental factors and relationships over time.
- Role-modeling and personal reflection may be the most important ways professionalism is taught; however, various teaching methods have been described.
- Assessing and remediating professionalism requires a range of approaches over time, and specific instruments are available.
- Faculty development and the clinical learning environment are critical to the successful teaching of professionalism.
- In the twenty-first century, e-professionalism, culture, diversity, equity and inclusion, structural competence, and interprofessional professionalism have become increasingly important topics in professionalism education in psychiatry.

# REFERENCES

Accreditation Council for Graduate Medical Education: 1999 Annual Report: Assuring the Quality of Medical Care. Chicago, IL, Accreditation Council for Graduate Medical Education, 1999. Available at: https://www.acgme.org/Portals/0/PDFs/an_1999AnnRep.pdf. Accessed December 5, 2019

Accreditation Council for Graduate Medical Education, American Board of Psychiatry and Neurology: The Psychiatry Milestone Project, July 2015. Available at: https://www.acgme.org/Portals/0/PDFs/Milestones/PsychiatryMilestones.pdf?ver=2015-11-06-120520-753. Accessed September 24, 2019.

Accreditation Council for Graduate Medical Education: Psychiatry Milestones, Second Revision, March 2020. Available at https://www.acgme.org/Portals/0/PDFs/Milestones/PsychiatryMilestones2.0.pdf?ver=2020-03-10-152105-537. Accessed November 23, 2020.

American Board of Internal Medicine Foundation, American College of Physicians–American Society of Internal Medicine Foundation, European Federation of Internal Medicine: Medical professionalism in the new millennium: a physicians charter. Ann Intern Med 136(3):243–246, 2002

Arnold L, Sullivan C, Quaintance J: Remediation of unprofessional behavior, in Teaching Medical Professionalism: Supporting the Development of a Professional Identity. Edited by Cruess RL, Cruess SR, Steinert Y. Cambridge, UK, Cambridge University Press, 2016, pp 169–185

Association of American Medical Colleges: Medical School Graduation Questionnaire: 2018 All Schools Summary Report. Washington, DC, Association of American Medical Colleges, July 2018. Available at: https://www.aamc.org/system/files/reports/1/2018gqallschoolssummaryreport.pdf. Accessed December 5, 2019.

Baernstein A, Fryer-Edwards K: Promoting reflection on professionalism: a comparison trial of educational interventions for medical students. Acad Med 78:742–747, 2003

Bagian JP, Weiss KB: The overarching themes from the CLER National Report of Findings. J Grad Med Educ 8(2 suppl 1):21–23, 2016

Bakker D, Kazantzis N, Rickwood D, Richard N: Mental health smartphone apps: review and evidence-based recommendations for future developments. JMIR Mental Health 1:3(1), 2016

Barry D, Cyran E, Anderson RJ: Common issues in medical professionalism: room to grow. Am J Med 108(2):136–142, 2000

Birden H, Glass N, Wilson I, et al: Teaching professionalism in medical education: a best evidence medical education (BEME) systematic review. BEME Guide No 25. Med Teach 35(7):e1252–e1266, 2013

Birden H, Glass N, Wilson I, et al: Defining professionalism in medical education: a systematic review. Med Teach 36(1):47–61, 2014

Boenink AD, de Jonge P, Smal K, et al: The effects of teaching medical professionalism by means of vignettes: an exploratory study. Med Teach 27:429–432, 2005

Bromage B, Encandela JA, Cranford M, et al: Understanding health disparities through the eyes of community members: a structural competency education intervention. Acad Psychiatry 43(2):244–247, 2019

Bursch BB, Placentini J, Cook IA, et al: Everyday mishaps and lapses in ethics, professionalism, and self-care: a faculty development workshop. Acad Psychiatry 40:97–99, 2016

Chretien KC, Greysen SR, Chretien JP, et al: Online posting of unprofessional content by medical students. JAMA 302(12):1309–1315, 2009

Cruess R, McIlroy JH, Cruess S, et al: The Professionalism Mini-Evaluation Exercise: a preliminary investigation. Acad Med 81(10 suppl):S74–S78, 2006

Cruess RL, Cruess SR, Boudreau D, et al: A schematic representation of the professional identity formation and socialization of medical students and residents: a guide for medical educators. Acad Med 90:718–725, 2015

Cruess RL, Cruess SR, Steinert Y: Amending Miller's pyramid to include professional identity formation. Acad Med 91(2):180–185, 2016a

Cruess RL, Cruess SR, Steinert Y (eds): Teaching Medical Professionalism: Supporting the Development of a Professional Identity, 2nd Edition. Cambridge, UK, Cambridge University Press, 2016b

DeJong SM: What is professionalism?, in Blogs and Tweets, Texting and Friending: Social Media and Online Professionalism in Health Care. San Diego, CA, Elsevier, 2014, pp 1–10

DeJong SM, Benjamin S, Anzia J, et al: Professionalism and the internet in psychiatry: what to teach and how to teach it. Acad Psychiatry 36(5):356–362, 2012

Dingle A, DeJong S, Madaan V, Ascherman L: Teaching ethics in child and adolescent psychiatry: vignette-based curriculum. MedEdPortal.org, June 17, 2016. Available at: https://www.mededportal.org/doi/10.15766/mep_2374-8265.10418. Accessed November 23, 2020

Edgar L, Roberts S, Holmboe E: Milestones 2.0: a step forward. J Grad Med Educ 10:367–369, 2018

Gabbard GO: Digital professionalism. Acad Psychiatry 43:259–263, 2019

Gabbard GO, Roberts LW, Crisp-Han H, et al: Professionalism in Psychiatry. Washington, DC, American Psychiatric Publishing, 2012

Greysen SR, Chretien KC, Kind T, et al: Physician violations of online professionalism and disciplinary actions: a national survey of state medical boards. JAMA 307(11):1141–1142, 2012

Gupta M, Forlini C, Lenton K, et al: The hidden ethics curriculum in two Canadian psychiatry residency programs: a qualitative study. Acad Psychiatry 40:592–599, 2016

Hafferty FW, Hafler JP: The hidden curriculum, structural disconnects, and the socialization of new professionals, in Extraordinary Learning in the Workplace. Edited by Hafler JP. Dordrecht, The Netherlands, Springer, 2011, pp 17–35

Hammick M, Freedth D, Copperman J, Goodsman D: Being Interprofessional. Cambridge, UK, Polity Press, 2009

Higginbotham EJ: Professionalism in the 21st century: challenges and opportunities, in Medical Professionalism Best Practices: Professionalism in the Modern Era. Edited by Byyny RL, Paauw DS, Papadakis M, Pfeil SA. Aurora, CO, Alpha Omega Alpha Honor Medical Society, 2017, pp 117–128

Hilty DM, Crawford A, Teshima J, et al: A framework for tele-psychiatric training and e-health: competency-based education, evaluation and implications. Int Rev Psychiatry 27(6):569–92, 2015

Hilty DM, Chan S, Torous J, et al: Mental health, smartphone/device, and apps for psychiatry and medicine: competencies, training and faculty development issues, in Professional Development for Psychiatrists. Psychiatr Clin North Am 42(3):513–534, 2019

Hodges BD, Ginsburg S, Cruess R, et al: Assessment of professionalism: recommendations from the Ottawa 2010 conference. Med Teach 33(5):354–363, 2011

Hodges LE, Tak HJ, Curlin FA, Yoon JD: Whistle-blowing in medical school: a national survey on peer accountability and professional misconduct in medical students. Acad Psychiatry 40:530–533, 2016

Hojat M, Mangione S, Nasca TJ, et al: The Jefferson scale of physician empathy: developmental and preliminary psychometric data. Educ Psychol Meas 61(2):349–365, 2001

Huckvale K, Torous J, Larsen ME: Assessment of the data-sharing and privacy practices of smartphone apps for depression and smoking cessation. JAMA Open Network 2(4):e192542, 2019

Humphrey HJ, Levinson D: The learner and the learning environment—a complex interaction, in Medical Professionalism Best Practices: Professionalism in the Modern Era. Edited by Byyny RL, Paauw DS, Papadakis M, Pfeil SA. Aurora, CO, Alpha Omega Alpha Honor Medical Society, 2017, pp 97–115

Institute of Medicine Committee on Understanding and Eliminating Racial and Ethnic Disparities in Health Care: Unequal Treatment: Confronting Racial and Ethnic Disparities in Health Care. Edited by Smedley BD, Stith AY, Nelson AR. Washington, DC, National Academies Press, 2003

Interprofessional Education Collaborative: Core Competencies for Interprofessional Collaborative Practice: Report of an Expert Panel. Washington, DC, Interprofessional Educational Collaborative, 2011. Available at: https://www.aacom.org/docs/default-source/insideome/ccrpt05-10-11.pdf?sfvrsn=77937f97_2. Accessed September 24, 2019.

Irby DM, Hamstra SJ: Parting the clouds: three professionalism frameworks in medical education. Acad Med 91:1606–1611, 2016

Irvine D: The performance of doctors: the new professionalism. Lancet 353:1174–1177, 1999

Jain S, Hoop JG, Dunn LB, et al: Psychiatry residents' attitudes on ethics and professionalism: multisite survey results. Ethics Behav 20:10–20, 2010

Jain S, Lapid MI, Dunn LB, Roberts LW: Psychiatric residents' need for education about informed consent, principles of ethics and professionalism, and caring for vulnerable populations: results of a multi-site survey. Acad Psychiatry 35:184–190, 2011

Kao A: Ethics, law and professionalism: what physicians need to know, in Measuring Medical Professionalism. Edited by Stern DT. New York, Oxford University Press, 2005, pp 366–370

Kesselheim JC, McMahon GT, Joffe S: Development of a test of residents' ethics knowledge for pediatrics (TREK-P). J Grad Med Educ 4(2):242–245, 2012

Kwan YW, Png K, Phang JK, et al: A systematic review of the quality and utility of observer-based instruments for assessing medical professionalism. J Grad Med Educ 10(6):628–638, 2018

Larsen ME, Huckvale K, Nicholas J, et al: Using science to sell apps: evaluation of mental health app store quality claims. NPH Digit Med 22:2–18, 2019

Lewis J, Allan S: Physician-patient boundaries: professionalism training using video vignettes. MedEdPortal.org, June 10, 2016. Available at: https://www.mededportal.org/doi/full/10.15766/mep_2374-8265.10412. Accessed November 23, 2020.

Liaison Committee on Medical Education: Functions and Structure of a Medical School: Standards for Accreditation of Medical Education Programs Leading to the M.D. Degree. Washington, DC, Liaison Committee on Medical Education, 2020. Available at: https://lcme.org/publications. Accessed November 23, 2020.

Liu HY, Beresin EV, Chisolm MS: Social media skills for professional development in psychiatry and medicine. Psychiatr Clin North Am 42(3):483–492, 2019

Maheu MM, Drude KP, Hertlein KM, et al: Correction to: An interdisciplinary framework for telebehavioral health competencies. J Technol Behav Sci 3:108–140, 2018

Marrero I, Bell M, Dunn LB, Roberts LW: Assessing professionalism and ethics knowledge and skills: preferences of psychiatric residents. Acad Psychiatry 37(6):392–397, 2013

Martinez W, Etchegary JM, Thomas EJ, et al: "Speaking up" about patient safety concerns and unprofessional behaviors among residents: validation of two scales. BMJ Qual Saf 24(11):671–680, 2015

Mavis B, Sousa A, Lipscomb W, Rappley MD: Learning about medical student mistreatment from responses to the medical school graduation questionnaire. Acad Med 89(5):705–711, 2014

McDaniel MA, Hartman NS, Whetzel DL, Grubb WL III: Situational judgment tests, response instructions and validity: a meta-analysis. Pers Psychol 60(1):63–91, 2007

McLachlan JC, Finn G, MacNaughton J: The conscientiousness index: a novel tool to explore students' professionalism. Acad Med 84(5):559–565, 2009

McLeary-Gaddy AT, Scales R: Addressing mental health stigma, implicit bias, and stereotypes in medical school. Acad Psychiatry 43(5):512–515, 2019

Miller GE: The assessment of clinical skills/competence/performance. Acad Med 65(9 suppl):S63–S67, 1990
Molleman E, Rink F: Professional identity formation among medical specialists. Med Teach 35(10):875–876, 2013
Moss J, Teshima J, Leszcz M: Peer group mentoring of junior faculty. Acad Psychiatry 32(3):230–235, 2008
Nath C, Schmidt R, Gunel E: Perceptions of professionalism vary most with educational rank and age. J Dent Educ 70(8):825–834, 2006
Norcini JJ, Shea JA: Assessment of professionalism and progress in the development of a professional identity, in Teaching Medical Professionalism: Supporting the Development of a Professional Identity. Edited by Cruess RL, Cruess SR, Steiner Y. Cambridge, UK, Cambridge University Press, 2016, pp 155–168
Nordquista J, Hall J, Caverzagie K, et al: The clinical learning environment. Med Teach 41(4):366–372, 2019
Paauw DS, Papadakis M, Pfeil S: Generational differences in the interpretation of professionalism, in Medical Professionalism Best Practices: Professionalism in the Modern Era. Edited by Byyny RL, Paauw DS, Papadakis M, Pfeil SA. Aurora, CO, Alpha Omega Alpha Honor Medical Society, 2017, pp 33–40
Papadakis MA, Teherani A, Banach MA, et al: Disciplinary action by medical boards and prior behavior in medical school. N Engl J Med 353:2673–2682, 2005
Plakiotis C: Programmatic assessment of professionalism in psychiatric education: a literature review and implementation guide. Adv Exp Med Biol 989:217–233, 2017
Rademacher R, Simpson D, Marcdante K: Critical incidents as a technique for teaching professionalism. Med Teach 32(3):244–249, 2010
Regan L, Hexom B, Nazario S, et al: Remediation methods for milestones related to interpersonal and communication skills and professionalism. J Grad Med Educ 8(1):18–23, 2016
Relman AS: Medical professionalism in the commercialized healthcare market. JAMA 298:2668–2670, 2007
Rider EA: Competency 6: professionalism, in A Practical Guide to Teaching and Assessing the ACGME Core Competencies. Edited by Rider EA, Nawotniak RH, Smith G. Marblehead, MA, HCPro, 2007, pp 189–236
Roberts LW, Green Hammond KA, Geppert CMA, Warner TD: The positive role of professionalism and ethics training in medical education: a comparison of medical student and resident perspectives. Acad Psychiatry 28:170–182, 2004
Rothman D: Medical professionalism: focusing on the real issues. N Engl J Med 342:1284–1286, 2000
Rougas S, Gentilesco B, Green E, Flores L: Twelve tips for addressing medical student and resident physician lapses in professionalism. Med Teach 37:901–907, 2015
Schnapp BH, Ritter D, Kraut AS, et al: Assessing residency applicants' communication and professionalism: standardized video interview scores compared to faculty gestalt. West J Emerg Med 20(1):132–137, 2019
Schuwirth L, van der Vleuten C, Durning SJ: What programmatic assessment in medical education can learn from healthcare. Perspect Med Educ 6:211–215, 2017
Soklaridis S, Lopez J, Charach N, et al: Developing a mentorship program for psychiatry residents. Acad Psychiatry 39(1):10–15, 2015

Steinert Y: Faculty development to support professionalism and professional identity formation, in Teaching Medical Professionalism: Supporting the Development of a Professional Identity. Edited by Cruess RL, Cruess SR, Steinert Y. Cambridge, UK, Cambridge University Press, 2016, pp 124–139

Stephenson AE, Adshead LE, Higgs RH: The teaching of professional attitudes within UK medical schools: reported difficulties and good practice. Med Educ 40:1072–1080, 2006

Swick HM: Viewpoint: professionalism and humanism beyond the academic health center. Acad Med 82:1022–1028, 2007

Ten Cate O: Trust, competence, and the supervisor's role in postgraduate training. BMJ 333:748–751, 2006

Thistlethwaite JE, Kumar K, Roberts C: Becoming interprofessional: professional identity formation in the health professions, in Teaching Medical Professionalism: Supporting the Development of a Professional Identity. Edited by Cruess RL, Cruess SR, Steinert Y. Cambridge, UK, Cambridge University Press, 2016, pp 140–154

Tucker C, Choby B, Moore A, et al: Teachers as learners: developing professionalism feedback skills via observed structured teaching encounters. Teach Learn Med 29(4):373–377, 2017

Van Zanten M, Boulet JR, Norcini JJ, McKinley D: Using a standardized patient assessment to measure professional attributes. Med Educ 39(1):20–29, 2005

Wagner P, Hendrich J, Moseley G, Hudson V: Defining medical professionalism: a qualitative study. Med Educ 41:288–294, 2007

Wear D, Zarconi J: Can compassion be taught? Let's ask our students. J Gen Intern Med 23:948–953, 2008

Weiss KB, Bagian JP, Nasca TJ: The clinical learning environment: the foundation of graduate medical education. JAMA 309(16):1687–1688, 2013

Woodruff JN, Angelos P, Valaitis S: Medical professionalism: one size fits all? Perspect Biol Med 51:525–534, 2008

# CHAPTER 3

# WELLNESS, BURNOUT, AND RESILIENCE

Joan M. Anzia, M.D.
Carol A. Bernstein, M.D.

**Residency** training has changed dramatically since the 1990s. The experiential "see one, do one, teach one" educational model has been replaced by increasingly rigorous models of graduate medical education that designate what curricula are included, how education should be measured and evaluated, and the types of outcomes required of graduates. The long-standing challenges in medical culture that contribute to stress, burnout, and depression are now actively being addressed by groups such as the Accreditation Council for Graduate Medical Education (ACGME), Association of American Medical Colleges (AAMC), American Medical Association (AMA), and National Academy of Medicine. In this chapter, we focus on training residents to develop adaptive expertise so they can enjoy fulfilling careers characterized by personal well-being as well as outstanding care for patients. The evidence for some interventions to enhance well-being is scarce; however, a strong, supportive, and responsive community, a sense that work is meaningful and important, and the presence of knowledgeable teachers and supervisors who provide guidance and timely interventions are all important protective elements for residents in training.

# HISTORY AND LITERATURE

Challenges to the mental health of physicians are not new. In 2003, the AMA convened experts from across medicine to understand challenges to physician mental health. In a consensus paper, they concluded that physicians accord low priority to their own mental health despite burdens of mental disorders and suicide (Center et al. 2003). The next decade brought little change, until the highly publicized deaths by suicide of two medical interns from two different programs in New York City within 5 days of each other in 2014.

At its scheduled board meeting that September, the ACGME reviewed those events, discussed similar deaths in other programs, and concluded that concerns about physician health were reaching epidemic proportions. A Task Force on Physician Wellbeing was formed, and, in conjunction with leadership from the AAMC, plans were made to hold a symposium to address the issue in the fall of 2015. Subsequently, leadership from the ACGME and the AAMC joined forces with the National Academy of Medicine and created the Action Collaborative on Clinician Wellbeing and Resilience. More than 200 organizations have signed on to this initiative as of this writing.

In 2019, in response to concerns about resident mental health and well-being, the ACGME significantly altered its common program requirements. The new requirements, in section VI.C, highlight the importance of resident well-being and programs' responsibility to monitor and foster well-being in trainees (Accreditation Council for Graduate Medical Education 2019). They emphasize a culture of safety that ensures the availability of counseling and treatment and attends to the well-being of the entire health care team:

> The responsibility of the program, in partnership with the Sponsoring Institution, to address well-being must include: efforts to enhance the meaning that each resident finds in the experience of being a physician, including protecting time with patients, minimizing non-physician obligations, providing administrative support, promoting progressive autonomy and flexibility, and enhancing professional relationships; attention to scheduling, work intensity, and work compression that impacts resident well-being; evaluating workplace safety data and addressing the safety of residents and faculty members; policies and programs that encourage optimal resident and faculty well-being. (Accreditation Council for Graduate Medical Education 2019)

Section VI.C specifically requires that residents be able to attend medical, dental, and mental health appointments during work hours if necessary, that the work environment be monitored for safety, and that support be provided after adverse events. It also states that residents must have time away from work for rest, exercise, and to spend with family and friends. It requires that programs monitor residents and faculty for burnout, depression, and substance abuse and establish ways to address such problems. Programs and sponsoring institutions must also educate residents and faculty members about the symptoms of burnout, depression, and substance abuse, as well as signs of fatigue. Programs and sponsoring institutions must ensure that residents have access to affordable, confidential mental assessment, counseling, and treatment at all times and that, when indicated, treatment be immediately available.

The medical literature has reported extensively on both burnout and mental health challenges among health care professionals and has highlighted these among trainees. Burnout rates are generally reported in the 60% range, and young physicians are increasingly concerned about the integration of work/life responsibilities. Sen et al. (2010) reported that rates of depression, as defined by Patient Health Questionnaire–9 scores >10, rise from a low of about 3% prior to the onset of training to approximately 25% within the first 3 months of internship and remain at that level throughout the internship year. Factors correlated with depression in residents include (but are not limited to) high levels of neuroticism, difficult early family environment, female gender, U.S. medical school training, higher mean work hours, and work/life conflict. Programs whose interns show higher levels of depression are characterized by longer work hours, less faculty involvement, poorer inpatient rotations, and a higher research score as measured by Doximity (Pereira-Lima et al. 2019). Most recently, studies have correlated long work hours and reduction of telomere length over the course of internship (Ridout et al. 2019). Other biomarkers and correlates have not yet been found.

Many studies in the literature show relationships between particular factors and increased reports of burnout and depressive and anxiety symptoms (Mata et al. 2015). *Burnout* generally has been described as a psychological condition characterized by depersonalization (feelings of cynicism and detachment), emotional exhaustion, and a sense of ineffectiveness and lack of accomplishment that emerge as a prolonged response to chronic job stressors (Maslach and Jackson 1981). Burnout in health care professionals has been linked to poorer patient care, more medical errors, dysfunctional relationships with colleagues, greater risks of substance abuse, depression and suicidal ideation, and a stronger intention to leave the medical profession. Drivers of burnout include excessive stress mediated by long hours, fatigue, work compression, and the intensity of the work environment; a loss of meaning in medicine and patient care; decreased support and increased responsibility along with a decrease in autonomy and flexibility; challenges in institutional cultures; a lack of professionalism; and problems with work/life integration. Other risk factors for burnout and distress include sleep deprivation; work being interrupted by personal concerns; high levels of anger, loneliness, or anxiety; the stress of work relationships; anxiety about competency; difficulty "unplugging" after work; and the regular use of alcohol and other drugs (Ey et al. 2013, 2016).

Although burnout and depression are not the same, their symptoms may be similar. Moreover, burnout may lead to depression in vulnerable individuals, and access to high-quality, timely, and low-cost mental health services is an essential part of any training program.

There has also been greater focus on the "epidemic" of suicide among trainees, although the rates of suicide are still lower than those in a control group of college graduates. Overall rates of suicide have been rising across the United States; it is difficult to know how much of this increase is due to increased recognition and greater awareness (Gold et al. 2013; Rubin 2014).

# DEVELOPMENTAL MODEL

Given all these issues, what are appropriate ways to think about burnout, developmental challenges, and mental health issues in the context of psychiatric training? We propose a developmental model of residency training that highlights typical challenges, transitions, and pivot points in education. We know that some common transitions in training are particularly vulnerable periods for trainees.

## After Recruitment and Match

In the weeks after Match results and graduation, many students use the break before the internship to travel and to spend time with family and friends. Some students may plan a wedding. This period is often a time of excitement, anticipation, and some anxiety, during which many will relocate. It is reassuring to incoming postgraduate year-1 (PGY1) residents to have regular contact with current residents in the program; this sets up expectations for a "buddy" program with identified senior residents who can answer questions and help the incoming PGY1 resident feel "part of the program family."

Some medical students arrive at residency with undisclosed histories of treatment for mood and anxiety disorders. Unfortunately, many of them stop medications before starting residency because their symptoms are well in remission by the end of medical school, because they do not want to be the "only" intern on psychotropic medications, or because they do not want to have to schedule appointments away from work. Medical students are also apprehensive about stigma regarding mental health treatment. Under the stress of internship, symptoms can recur and significantly affect the trainee's well-being. To prevent or minimize these events, some graduate medical education programs send a letter of congratulations after the Match that includes strong encouragement to continue with medical and mental health treatment during training and a list of available physicians near the hospital or medical center.

The literature is clear that life transitions also increase the risk of depression and suicide. Following the excitement of graduation and of finally "becoming a doctor," incoming house staff may experience stress in moving, separation from friends and families, and a postcelebration "letdown." Some institutions provide "opt-in" sessions with mental health counselors for incoming trainees for such reasons. Whether this practice alleviates some of the stressors and reduces the reluctance to seek treatment down the road if symptoms persist remains unclear.

## New Postgraduate Year 1 and Well-Being

### *ORIENTATION*

The new class has arrived, and PGY1 residents are generally excited and eager. Programs, departments, and institutional communities that feel welcoming are protective for new trainees, so get-togethers and celebrations are very important. Many chairs and program directors host welcome events at their homes and include interns' significant others (who are generally a major support for the intern). Beginning PGY1 residents need to feel that they are valued and included and that the program will "have their backs" as they navigate their internship year.

Orientation is one of the most important events of the intern year. Interns are both excited and anxious, so they likely will remember only some of the content taught. What is most important is that they are given the program directors' and chief residents' cellphone numbers and told that they can and should call with any serious concerns or problems, day or night. In addition to other information, new residents should attend presentations on staying well during training, including practical topics such as

- Getting enough sleep, especially on night rotations (e.g., having room-darkening shades or curtains at home is important for day sleeping)
- Maintaining hydration and healthy food intake both day and night

- The importance of regular exercise and how to find time for it
- Symptoms of common illnesses and when to stay home from work
- How to prepare for call and night float (including assembling a night float backpack with water bottle, snacks, toiletries)
- The importance of maintaining contact with family, friends, and peers during training
- What to do if they become ill or too fatigued on night float or call
- The symptoms of fatigue and how to mitigate it

One aspect of orientation that is gaining favor among programs is to provide a separate orientation for residents' spouses and significant others, including close friends. In many cases, the stress of internship will be evident first in their home environment. Alerting interns' support community to some of the challenges and helping them understand the nature of the intern work experience will make it easier for that community to provide support and intervene if necessary.

PGY1 residents should also learn the symptoms and signs of burnout and depression during internship and residency and be strongly encouraged, should they develop symptoms, to make contact with mental health resources provided by the institution. Residents should be informed that they can and should attend any medical or mental health appointments during the work day, after giving notice to their attending physician. Faculty members should also understand that residents must be able to leave rotations during the work day to attend these appointments. The program director must ensure that residents are able to attend appointments during rotations without fear of repercussions from a rotation supervisor (even a division chief or department chair).

### *ROTATIONS OUTSIDE OF PSYCHIATRY*

One challenge for program directors and chief residents is staying connected with PGY1 interns who are on medicine, pediatrics, family medicine, and neurology rotations. In order to monitor the interns' progress and well-being, psychiatry program directors should develop and maintain relationships and lines of communication with the program directors in those specialties to discuss how their interns are faring. Program directors should plan regular outreach to the interns, and chiefs should plan regular evening social events where interns on other specialty rotations can join fellow psychiatry residents. If an intern is struggling on nonpsychiatry rotations, the psychiatry program director, in collaboration with the specialty program director, should meet with that intern to evaluate for any depression, anxiety, professionalism, or learning problems and to provide support or other targeted intervention.

At times, the psychiatry program director may learn about stressors on a medicine or neurology rotation that can contribute to burnout or depression. For example, a psychiatry PGY1 resident is assigned more on-call shifts than pediatrics residents on the same rotation or is assigned to the most demanding neurology unit for their entire 2-month rotation. Ideally, program directors should prevent such occurrences by careful planning with the other specialty program director, but if rotation problems do develop, the psychiatry program director must respond quickly. The PGY1 resident may be subjected to harassment from a nonpsychiatrist attending physician who disparages psychiatry. In such situations, the psychiatry program director must act quickly and decisively to either remedy the stressor or move the resident to another rotation.

It is important to remember the power differential between attending physicians and PGY1 residents; the program director must ensure that residents are not being subjected to unrealistic service expectations, hazing, demeaning comments, or harassment, which are all contributors to burnout. Not infrequently, psychiatric residents rotate on other services at later points in the academic year after spending 6 months on the psychiatry service. As a result, they may appear to be "behind" fellow nonpsychiatry interns who have been working longer in medicine, pediatrics, and neurology. The program director should gently remind colleagues in other departments of this fact and recommend that the psychiatry interns be given an orientation to the service and additional support early in the rotation.

## Common Work Struggles of PGY1 Residents

### *TIME MANAGEMENT*

A primary challenge for residents in PGY1 is time management. Medical students frequently set their own schedule, and students may have flexibility even during clerkships. This all changes when residents are responsible for patient care and prioritizing and efficiency become very important.

### *UNCERTAINTY ABOUT SPECIALTY CHOICE*

With the disappearance of traditional "transitional year" programs and the growing preponderance of 3-year medical schools, students have diminished opportunities to truly interact with a variety of specialties. Specialty choices are frequently determined by clerkship experiences (the number-one factor noted on the AAMC graduation questionnaire) and by exposure to dynamic faculty. As a result, when trainees move into internship, questions about their career choice may emerge. It is not uncommon for one or two interns in a class to contemplate or decide to switch to another specialty. Doubts about specialty choice can contribute to anxiety and unhappiness in the intern year.

*ANXIETY ABOUT NIGHT CALL*

In some programs, an intern's first exposure to psychiatry may be night call, frequently in an emergency setting. Isolation, concerns about competency, and sleep deprivation may contribute to stress, burnout, and depression. Programs should make every effort to maintain close contact with PGY1 residents during their on-call experiences and to ensure that they have appropriate orientation and support.

## Postgraduate Year 2

For many house staff, the beginning of PGY2 represents a "return to what I came here to do"; they are relieved and happy to be working in psychiatry after an initial period of training in other specialties. On the flip side, PGY2 may increase anxiety for residents who feel they have to "prove themselves" now that they are in their chosen profession. In addition, most programs have PGY2 rotations that are heavily inpatient. Psychiatric hospitalization is now reserved for acutely ill patients, who are briefly admitted for stabilization and triage. Seriously ill patients precipitate a range of responses in residents, from fear to overidentification. Moreover, many programs deal with the on-call experience via night float rotations, which has many advantages, but residents often feel isolated and disconnected from their peers and the training program while on night float. In addition, residents may fear they are missing out on important learning experiences during the day. Video recording lectures and developing peer support to mitigate against isolation during night float may help. Forming "process" or "Balint" groups as part of the curriculum to address some of the stresses of becoming a psychiatrist may enhance well-being for all trainees.

## Postgraduate Year 3

In many programs, PGY3 transitions residents from the "cocoon" of inpatient rotations to settings in which they are primarily treating patients independently. These experiences increase autonomy and may be overwhelming for residents who worry about their competency and about adverse patient outcomes, such as suicide. Relationships with faculty are particularly critical in the outpatient year. If the resident/faculty pairing is not optimal, it may create additional stress for the resident. In addition, events such as patient suicide may complicate a resident's sense of mastery and contribute to increased anxiety, stress, and depression.

Residents applying to child psychiatry in PGY3 may feel burdened by the process and struggle to maintain a strong sense of connection to the program and their colleagues as they work through the separation process, particularly just prior to transfer.

## Postgraduate Year 4

PGY4 is a time for consolidation of skills and feelings of accomplishment. In most programs, residents work in a supervisory capacity and may work call shifts from home. Rotations include electives in which residents are free to pursue areas of interest. This change from "requirements" is usually liberating, but it may be offset by concerns about fellowship decisions, employment, and the loss of camaraderie that the end of training signifies. "Leaving the nest" may trigger the ambivalence that all children feel when leaving home, and residents may experience increased distress. Many programs hold "transition to practice" seminars to help ease the anxiety of completing training, in which faculty can discuss career planning, the job search, future work/life integration, financial planning, and termination with patients, faculty supervisors, peers, and the program.

## Adverse Clinical Events

Medical literature describes the deep impact that adverse clinical events often have on the well-being of physicians, particularly residents. Physician and trainee distress in the aftermath of such an event includes increased anxiety about future errors, negative impact on confidence, negative impact on sleep, and reduced job satisfaction. The "worst outcome" in psychiatry is generally a patient's suicide. Unfortunately, between 20% and 60% of residents experience a patient suicide during training; these are more likely to occur when a resident is on acute care services (Fang et al. 2007). Multiple studies describe the range of reactions that residents experience in the aftermath of a suicide. The usual progression begins with shock and numbness and a feeling that the death is not real, followed by high anxiety and concerns about having "missed something" or made an error in assessment, treatment, or disposition. The resident is tempted to go over chart notes repeatedly, trying to understand what went wrong. Anxiety is accompanied by grief and sadness over the loss of the patient and for the patient's family. Residents can feel a significant loss of confidence, even to the point of wondering whether they are fit to be in psychiatry; they may feel like imposters and think that their colleagues and supervisors view them as less than competent.

Most residents have difficulty sleeping for a night or more following an adverse event and may be in a state of sympathetic hyperarousal. For some, these symptoms do not resolve without treatment. Physicians, including trainees, commonly become more risk averse in the aftermath of an adverse event and attempt to avoid exposure to similar patients or procedures. Considerable shame is common and leads to a tendency to isolate and not seek support. Physicians and residents also struggle with concerns about malpractice vis-à-vis discussing the event with peers or supervisors.

Program directors have a number of crucial tasks in the aftermath of such events:

1. They must be notified immediately by the rotation director or the faculty supervisor about any adverse event and must personally inform every resident who worked with the patient. In addition to sharing facts about the event, they should express their condolences and support residents through the range of reactions that follow.
2. They should assess residents' level of distress and describe and normalize some of the common experiences following such events, such as difficulty sleeping.
3. They should consider offering residents some time to reflect and inquire what would be most helpful. Most residents prefer to stay with peers rather than take the rest of the day off; they think that going home is somehow associated with "having done something wrong." Residents vary in their preference.
4. They should check in briefly each day with residents regarding sleep, mood, and overall functioning for a few days after the event and at the 1-week anniversary.
5. If a critical incident review or a morbidity and mortality conference is to be held, they should meet with residents beforehand to explain the process and purpose and should attend with the residents.

The immediate aftermath of such adverse events is often a harried and emotionally charged time, so formal policies that describe how residents are notified about a patient's suicide and the role of the program director are extremely helpful.

## Managing Life Events That Can Affect Well-Being

PGY1 residents generally have little idea how to manage their obligations as a physician and address their personal or family issues. They will need active guidance and support from program directors to learn the principles of handling these often complex situations. Several examples of such situations follow.

A program director received an early Sunday-morning phone call from one of his PGY1 residents. The resident was in the emergency department of a community hospital and had been told that he needed an appendectomy. He asked the program director if he should request a transfer to the teaching hospital so he could "be closer to his patients on the inpatient unit." The program director told the resident that he absolutely must stay where he was and have the surgery. The resident then stated that he would be back at work within 2 days. The program director (with some humor) responded that no, that would not happen, and that the resident needed to be off for at least a week and should only return when cleared by the surgeon.

A PGY1 resident 2 months into training called her program director. The new condo she and her husband had moved into had been severely damaged by a fire and was uninhabitable. She felt overwhelmed and was unsure if it was expected that she attend her emergency medicine rotation that day. The program director advised her that her first priorities were her safety and that of her family and finding a new temporary home and told her that she would need at least a week away to take care of those immediate needs. The program director then called the program director of emergency medicine to explain the situation and plan for ongoing communication. The program director provided support with other practical matters, and the resident's classmates provided material and emotional support.

As difficult as life situations such as these during residency may be, they offer program directors the opportunity to model and teach residents how to balance responsibilities as a physician with principles of self-care. There is no written manual to teach how to navigate these events. Because every event is unique, the necessary tools are principles, values, and a model for thoughtful decision making. Such real-life lessons help residents build a foundation of adaptive expertise for making future difficult decisions. In the program community, resident peers will also likely learn how the program director and affected residents manage the event and learn these principles as well as the importance of peer support.

### *MARRIAGE*

In the not-so-distant past, residents tended to plan weddings before they started residency or in the last year of training, when schedules are more flexible. Currently, residents commonly marry throughout residency training. PGY1 residents are often unaware of the potential stressors of planning a wedding while navigating call shifts and the other physical, cognitive, and emotional demands of early training. It may help to address this subject during PGY1 orientation and provide information about available vacation time and delegating wedding planning tasks, as well as highlighting the primacy of self-care.

Family reunions, friends' weddings, and other positive events can present challenges. Often, PGY1 is the first time a resident has to make difficult choices between the commitment to medicine and personal freedom, and family and friends may not understand the choice to not be present. Such experiences help residents build adaptive expertise in making future choices.

#### *CHILDBEARING AND CHILDREARING*

Resident pregnancies may be a source of anticipation, joy, and celebration in a program, but they also entail adjustments to rotation and call schedules that can be challenging. A healthy pregnant resident usually manages work and her pregnant status well and without undue stress. However, she may struggle with guilt about the need for fellow residents to cover her patients while she is on maternity leave. The program director should relieve these guilt feelings and manage any negative reactions from the resident group, such as covert envy or resentment.

#### *MEDICAL ILLNESS AND MENTAL HEALTH CHALLENGES*

Although generally rare, medical or mental health issues may arise that necessitate a resident leave of absence. Maintaining privacy for the resident while simultaneously dealing with coverage challenges can be a particularly thorny problem. Programs benefit from having explicit policies and procedures that describe exactly how such situations are handled and what impact a resident's leave time will have on completion of training. Reviewing these processes often should minimize the disruptive impact on both the program and the resident. A resident suicide or suicide attempt will have a profound impact on the entire community and is beyond the scope of this chapter; the American Foundation for Suicide Prevention publication *After a Suicide: A Toolkit for Physician Residency/Fellowship Programs* (Dyrbye et al. 2018) is an invaluable resource for such an event.

## CONCLUSION

In summary, residency training is a time of both great opportunity and significant challenges. Creating a training environment that optimizes learning, development, growth, and camaraderie goes a long way toward providing trainees with a solid foundation for their future careers.

## — KEY POINTS —

- Burnout, depression, and suicide are common among physicians, and younger physicians are more at risk. Mandates to attend to faculty and resident wellness and mental health are now a part of Accreditation Council for Graduate Medical Education requirements.
- Program directors may enhance resilience and well-being by attending to developmental risks for stress over the residency trajectory.

# REFERENCES

Accreditation Council for Graduate Medical Education: Section VI.C., in Common Program Requirements (Residency). Chicago, IL, Accreditation Council for Graduate Medical Education, July 2019. Available at: https://www.acgme.org/Portals/0/PFAssets/ProgramRequirements/CPRResidency2019.pdf. Accessed July 1, 2020.

Center C, Davis M, Detre T, et al: Confronting depression and suicide in physicians: a consensus statement. JAMA 289(23):3161–3166, 2003

Dyrbye L, Konopasek L, Moutier C: After a Suicide: A Toolkit for Physician Residency/Fellowship Programs. New York, American Foundation for Suicide Prevention, 2018. Available at: http://www.acgme.org/portals/0/pdfs/13287_afsp_after_suicide_clinician_toolkit_final_2.pdf. Accessed July 1, 2020.

Ey S, Moffit M, Kinzie JM, et al: If you build it, they will come: attitudes of medical residents and fellows about seeking services in a resident wellness program. J Grad Med Educ 5(3):486–492, 2013

Ey S, Moffit M, Kinzie JM, Brunette PH: Feasibility of a comprehensive wellness and suicide prevention program: a decade of caring for physicians in training and practice. J Grad Med Educ 8(5):747–753, 2016

Fang F, Kemp J, Jawandha A, et al.: Encountering patient suicide: a resident's experience. Acad Psychiatry 31:340–344, 2007

Gold KJ, Sen SA, Schwenk TL: Details on suicide among US physicians: data from the National Violent Death Reporting System. Gen Hosp Psychiatry 35(1):45–49, 2013

Maslach C, Jackson SE: The measurement of experienced burnout. J Occupat Behav 2:99–113, 1981

Mata DA, Ramos MA, Bansal N, et al: Prevalence of depression and depressive symptoms among resident physicians: a systematic review and meta-analysis. JAMA 314(22):2373–2383, 2015

Pereira-Lima K, Gupta R, Guille C, Sen S: Residency program factors associated with depressive symptoms in internal medicine interns: a prospective cohort study. Acad Med 94(6):869–875, 2019

Ridout KK, Ridout SJ, Guille C, et al: Physician-training stress and accelerated cellular aging. Biol Psychiatry 86(9):725–730, 2019
Rubin R: Recent suicides highlight need to address depression in medical students and residents. JAMA 312(17):1725–1727, 2014
Sen S, Kranzler HR, Krystal JH, et al: A prospective cohort study investigating factors associated with depression during medical internship. Arch Gen Psychiatry 67(6):557–565, 2010

# CHAPTER 4

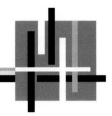

# MENTORING AND SUPERVISION

Donna M. Sudak, M.D.
Sallie G. DeGolia, M.D., M.P.H.

**Supervision** is essential to the education of psychiatrists, serving at least two critical functions. First is the ongoing educational preceptorship required in all graduate medical education. Second is the particular type of supervision that has a long tradition in the education of psychotherapists. Each has a vital educational role in psychiatric training.

Despite the significant place accorded supervision in training, an actual empirical basis for the practice is lacking. In fact, the most effective practices involved in training supervisors and supervising residents remain unclear. There is an emerging literature regarding the impact of supervision on therapist adherence and competence and patient outcomes in psychotherapy (see Milne and Reiser 2017) that validates the investment in this time-intensive process. As more research clarifies best training practices for supervisors, more supervisor trainings will materialize, resulting in an increase in effective supervision. Many therapist training organizations (e.g., the Academy of Cognitive Therapy, the British Association of Cognitive and Behavioral Psychotherapy) consider supervisor training and accreditation sufficiently important to create a separate specialty area of focus and attention in their accrediting standards.

Our aim in this chapter is to give an overview of evidence-informed supervisory practices and discuss specific concerns relating to boundaries and mentorship. Although the focus of this chapter is on supervision as conducted in psychotherapy training, the educational principles involved should generalize to supervision in other contexts in psychiatric education.

## KEY COMPONENTS OF PSYCHOTHERAPY SUPERVISION

### Building the Relationship

Supervision is learning that occurs in the context of a relationship. This makes it ideally suited to the skillset of psychiatrists because it parallels the psychotherapeutic process. The initial meetings of supervisor and supervisee should address both the relational needs of the dyad and the educational imperatives at hand. Several early behaviors of the supervisor facilitate a strong collaborative bond. First, supervisors should obtain sufficient information about their supervisees' background, prior clinical and didactic experience, current clinical assignment, and past experience with supervision in order to identify their educational needs. Supervision frequently entails an evaluative component that may have bearing on residents' promotion or employment; this feature may potentially interfere with trust and connection, so transparency about the evaluation process is extremely important. Warmth, interest, genuineness, and positive regard encourage residents to honestly exchange information and ideas (Bernard and Goodyear 2019; Shanfield et al. 1992). The supervisor must cultivate an atmosphere of mutual respect and trust to empower residents to share any aspects of patient care that may not be going well or that are a source of confusion or anxiety. Studies of supervision reveal that nondisclosure of difficult material in supervision is a significant problem and may adversely impact both patient care and the learning process (Ladany 2004). Managing residents' anxiety is critical to facilitate learning. Good supervisors foster a learning environment that excites residents about the process of curious inquiry and self-evaluation essential to therapist growth. The most effective supervisors develop a relationship in which residents can safely wrestle with difficult clinical questions and determine solutions independently; undue concern about negative evaluation will hamper this process.

Another important aspect of the supervisory alliance that requires careful consideration is managing ruptures. Supervisors must directly address any problems that arise and attempt to collaboratively develop a plan to solve them.

## Educational Goal Setting

After establishing the relationship, supervisors should assess residents' learning needs and help them set goals. A needs assessment should identify gaps in knowledge and promote excitement about supervision. The relationship is designed to help residents be more effective psychotherapists/psychiatrists. Setting goals has been recognized as a key component of improving performance (Milne and Reiser 2017). In psychiatry training, goal setting is complicated for three reasons. First, residents frequently begin psychotherapy supervision with limited knowledge and skills in any form of psychotherapy. They truly "don't know what they don't know." Until these skills are acquired, residents may have a limited capacity to reflect and may benefit less from Socratic questioning that facilitates independent practice. Second, residents are often extremely reluctant to admit gaps in their knowledge. The culture of medical training frequently employs shame as a training strategy (ineffective as it may be) when a resident does not know an answer. Such punishing experiences may result in residents who avoid admitting limitations or knowledge deficiencies and, therefore, will negatively impact well-intended supervision. The third challenge to goal setting is that residency requirements generally are not optional. Residents may have a negative view of requirements, and supervisors must work to promote receptivity.

In residency, defining learning goals may be easier when supervisors are familiar with the didactic training provided, Accreditation Council for Graduate Medical Education requirements, expectations listed on evaluation forms, and patient care opportunities at particular training sites. Supervisors must identify the explicit program or clinic learning goals if these are unclear and understand the particular clinical context in which residents are working. Supervisors should determine whether their residents have had experience that relates to the learning task at hand, such as prior experience in providing psychotherapy, and what the residents understand about the role and responsibility of each party in supervision.

Collaborative learning goals should be developed in the form of specific, well-defined units of performance that are easy to quantify and measure. Learning goals let residents know what they should master, guide supervisors in planning the instructional process, and provide both supervisors and residents a basis for evaluation. Setting learning goals should provide a framework for lifelong learning regarding how to approach a novel clinical problem.

## The Fine Print

Finally, we recommend writing a supervisory contract to clarify boundaries, expectations, and responsibilities. Such a contract should include the framework of supervision (e.g., frequency, time of meetings, contact numbers), any expectations, and the frequency of written assignments or recordings of patient sessions, as well as the plan for formal evaluation and feedback. The contract should specify the legal responsibilities of the supervisor, the patients for which the supervisor will be responsible, and the protocol for contacting the supervisor about patient emergencies. It is not unusual in residency for psychotherapy supervisors to not be the "supervisor of record," particularly if they are voluntary faculty or nonpsychiatrists. Therefore, an additional psychiatrist (generally someone on the faculty or based at the outpatient clinic site) may be responsible for reviewing documentation and for patient care emergencies; the supervisory contract must clearly spell out such arrangements.

In the early stages of supervision, residents may benefit from practicing how to explain to patients that their care will be discussed in supervision and how their confidentiality will be preserved. Residents may also need to roleplay how to obtain a patient's permission to record sessions. Roleplaying these discussions helps allay anxiety, builds skills and confidence, and provides a window into residents' basic interpersonal skill set.

## Supervision as an Educational Tool

Once the resident and supervisor have defined the terms of their relationship, they can begin working. For many supervisors, a "fresh take" on supervision is in order because many of us have been supervised with a "see one, do one, teach one" ethos. Traditionally, supervision consists of the supervisor listening to the resident describe a patient presentation (sometimes for at least half of the supervision time), entertaining questions, and telling the resident what to do. We believe this model is problematic on multiple levels. First, if the supervisor knows the resident is capable of assessment and case presentation (which should be determined at the start of supervision), spending supervision time performing such activities has limited utility. Instead, residents should be instructed to provide a written case summary to the supervisor for review prior to each session. Second, residents should be instructed how to formulate good questions for supervision. This process embodies the reflective attitude that is ideal for future growth and performance improvement. Third, "telling the resident what to do" actually decreases learning; we want residents to develop the capacity to think for themselves and to approach patients with a reflective attitude that will continue throughout their practice life. When residents reach a "stuck point," supervision should help them generate and evaluate solutions with increasing independence. Such a process often requires a great deal of deftness. First, the clinical situation must not be so urgent as to require immediate action; the supervisor must be more directive if time and efficiency are essential. Residents must have optimal levels of curiosity (think Goldilocks) to motivate further exploration. Additionally, if skills are not present, the supervisor must teach them. This delicate balance of inquiry, reflection, and instruction is one that the best supervisors keep at the front of their mind.

A second instructional imperative is to use multiple methods of instruction. Reflective questioning, roleplay, watching recorded materials, reviewing transcripts, diagramming vicious circles, encouraging deliberate practices, and other, more experiential modes of instruction enhance engagement in supervision. Experiential learning increases excitement. Learning is more effective if residents work on a patient problem that involves an emotional charge. Psychiatry is a difficult and emotionally taxing career. Residents who discuss patients about whom they have discomfort or anxiety more likely benefit from supervision and learn something important. Supervisors may model skills that help residents learn equanimity when managing difficult patients. Furthermore, cultivating reflective practices has been identified as a key element of successful development as a therapist (Bennett-Levy et al. 2003). Supervisors should model and encourage reflective practices and assign self-practice and self-reflection exercises.

## Evaluation and Feedback

Finally, evaluation and feedback are critical functions of supervision but are often fraught with difficulty from the perspective of both parties. Direct observation of skills either with roleplay or, preferably, by evaluating recordings or observing patient care is necessary to provide accurate and constructive feedback (Dorsey et al. 2018). Formative feedback is most effective when done collaboratively: first encouraging residents to self-assess and then developing an action plan based on areas identified for improvement. Effective feedback incorporates praise for what residents execute effectively and specifies behaviors that they need to improve. Precise feedback is most easily developed when the supervisor takes careful notes. Metrics that help the supervisor evaluate particular target behaviors (e.g., the Cognitive Therapy Rating Scale) also improve feedback. Opportunities to model and practice skills on the spot allow feedback to be integrated immediately. Activities that extend the learning across the week that follows are critical to make desired changes stick.

One special consideration is providing feedback in group supervision. Group supervision with embedded formative feedback may be a powerful learning experience, but many residents find receiving feedback in groups to be highly anxiety provoking. Thus, it is important to provide this feedback in a sensitive manner and to avoid any shaming of group members. Group norms regarding feedback from other members should be clarified at the outset.

Summative feedback should occur after careful preparation by both parties and must address strengths and areas for future growth. If the framework for the supervisory relationship has been carefully set, the resident will have reviewed the forms to be used for such feedback and prepared a self-assessment based on these criteria prior to such meetings. If group supervision is being conducted, any summative feedback should be given individually. When corrective feedback is extensive or relates to problematic behavior, it is wise to contact the training director and other members of the educational administration to discuss how best to proceed. Evaluating residents and managing problems are discussed in Chapter 13.

## MENTORING IN SUPERVISION

Mentorship may occur within supervision whenever a supervisor takes a personal interest in the supervisee's overall professional growth and development (Johnson 2007). One of the many potential roles of a psychiatry supervisor, mentorship is supported by clinical mental health supervision guidelines (Association for Counselor Education and Supervision 2016; Falender and Shafranske 2004).

How often mentorship develops within psychiatric supervision remains unclear. Mentorship is often seamlessly woven into the fabric of supervision. One qualitative study of faculty and resident trainees in an outpatient psychiatry clinic suggested that an interest in mentorship may differ between faculty and residents, particularly given a resident's developmental stage (Newman et al. 2016). Laschober et al. (2013) observed that clinical supervisors were more likely to engage in mentorship if they perceived fewer relationship costs with their trainee (e.g., disagreements, personality clashes, competitiveness) and greater benefits based on relationship quality (e.g., positive experience, trusted ally).

Well-documented benefits to mentoring include an increase in career guidance, networking, scholarly productivity, personal develop-

**Table 4–1.** Topics for mentorship

| |
|---|
| Identify personal values in the context of a career |
| Career and personal development |
| How to become involved in one's profession |
| How to engage in scholarship |
| How to negotiate positions |
| How to navigate administrative obstacles |
| How to recognize and manage complex political dynamics within one's training environment |
| How to balance personal and professional life |
| How to manage finances |
| How to pursue lifelong learning |

ment (Sambunjak et al. 2006), professional confidence and competence, satisfaction with training (Clark et al. 2000; Kaslow and Mascaro 2007), job satisfaction, higher academic self-efficacy (Feldman et al. 2010), and a decrease in tension between professional and personal conflicts (Laschober et al. 2013). Given these benefits, we discuss how to incorporate mentorship in supervision and avoid potential pitfalls.

Effective mentorship skills mirror those of a good supervisor: being empathic, respectful, learner centered, and an active listener and promoting the learner's development (Harms et al. 2019; Jackson et al. 2003; Koopman and Thiedke 2005; Shanfield et al. 1992; Stenfors-Hayes et al. 2011; Straus et al. 2009; Williams et al. 2004). At the beginning of supervision, the supervisor might introduce mentoring in the supervision contract and proactively include mentorship topics, such as those listed in Table 4–1.

Role modeling plays an important role in mentorship within supervision (Barnett 2011; Newman et al. 2016; Vasquez 1992). Through modeling ethical behaviors, supervisors help trainees learn to make reasoned and thoughtful decisions, avoid exploitations of self and others, promote independence, and ensure self-care (Barnett and Molzon 2014). Supervisors may also model self-directed learning.

The supervisor-mentor may advocate on behalf of the resident to ensure adequate learning resources, time for supervision, or professional development. If the supervisor observes significant stress or burnout in the resident, the supervisor might encourage the resident to consider ways to mitigate pressures and obtain help. If a resident's condition is of particular concern, the supervisor may need to inform program leadership to secure appropriate support. As an advocate, supervisors may actively promote their trainee-residents' career, inform them of professional meetings and conferences, introduce them to colleagues who will help with professional networking, invite them to co-author a publication or to collaborate on a research project, or ask them to serve on a professional committee or join a professional organization (Barnett and Molzon 2014; Johnson 2007). Although these actions may be perceived as boundary crossings (see next section), when executed intentionally and with careful monitoring, such behaviors may be acceptable.

Challenges involving mentorship in supervision are real, however; mentorship occurs more often within a positive supervisory relationship, so supervisors must manage interpersonal conflicts to avoid jeopardizing this possibility. It is incumbent on supervisors to safeguard against exploiting the inherent power differential in the supervisory relationship, such as by appropriating a resident's idea, withholding authorship, harassing a resident in any way (Fulton 2013; Kilgallon and Thompson 2012), or failing to fulfill an agreed-upon mentorship task. Furthermore, a supervisor may learn confidential information about a resident within the context of an imperfectly "secure" relationship and without reciprocal sharing. This lack of confidentiality exists by virtue of the supervisor's mandated role as evaluator; supervisors not only are charged with providing summative assessments to the training program but also may need to break confidentiality if a trainee's performance deficits fail to respond to repeated feedback or if the trainee presents a concern about fitness for duty or personal safety. It is the duty of the supervisor to inform the training program of such issues, preferably after communicating with the resident. The limits to supervisory confidentiality should be outlined at the start of supervision, even though the disclosure may lead to inadvertent negative consequences on the quality of that supervision.

Overall, mentorship is a highly valued part of trainee supervision. Creating a strong supervisory alliance and encouraging residents to take advantage of mentoring within the context of supervision may lead them to important and significant opportunities.

## BOUNDARIES WITHIN SUPERVISION

A supervisor's primary concern for the patient *and* the resident should align with the Hippocratic Oath: Do no harm. The best interests of the learner should be the utmost concern to the supervisor. Maintaining boundaries within supervision is equally as critical as within psychotherapy and is a fundamental responsibility of the supervisor. Boundaries form the ground rules of professional relationships.

Boundaries can be avoided, crossed, or violated. To identify a boundary encroachment in supervision, one must determine whether the behavior conforms to existing professional standards and whether the behavior is motivated by a desire to meet the needs of the resident or to meet the needs of the supervisor (Barnett and Molzon 2014). Some definitions include whether the behavior is welcomed by the trainee; this approach is complicated because a trainee may not recognize a boundary crossing or violation (Ellis et al. 2014) or may not be aware of its impact at the time.

Gutheil and Gabbard (1993) differentiated *boundary crossings* from *violations* within the context of psychotherapy. These definitions may apply to supervision. *Violations* are harmful, unethical, and are never appropriate, whereas *crossings* may or may not be problematic depending on the context. Boundary transgressions develop when a supervisor puts personal interests above those of a trainee. An important concept regarding boundaries is the "slippery slope," defined as breaks from the usual frame that may "crescendo" into increasing intrusions and culminate in an extreme violation, such as sexual contact (Gutheil and Gabbard 1993). Examples of boundary transgressions are listed in Table 4–2.

When supervisors neglect boundaries within supervision, trainees may feel responses ranging from uncomfortable or confused to exploited and harmed. Inappropriate crossings and violations may impair trainee learning and decrease disclosure (Mehr et al. 2010); increase a perception of multicultural incompetence (Singh and Chun 2010); lead to feelings of self-doubt, powerlessness, and fear; damage trust; increase stress; impair the trainee's professional or personal life; and affect the trainee's physical health (Nelson and Friedlander 2001). Boundary transgressions may also harm the educational environment, as in the case of a supervisor dating a trainee (Recupero et al. 2005). At this time, most training programs prohibit such behavior between a trainee and a supervisor. However, if a faculty member serving as a supervisor within the training program dates a resident who has *not* been their trainee, that resident is inadvertently and potentially placed in an unfairly "favored" position compared with peers. For example, other trainees may be excluded from informal relationships with other faculty that the "favored" resident forms as a result of the relationship or be excluded from educational opportunities only available to this resident.

The prevalence of boundary crossings or violations in supervision is unclear. Recupero et al. (2005) surveyed 154 residents (102 respondents) at four hospitals associated with an academic medical center, 25% of whom were psychiatry residents. Despite American Association of University Professors standards of conduct, many reported behaviors were

**Table 4–2.** Boundary transgressions

| | |
|---|---|
| Inappropriate self-disclosures | Asking a trainee out on a date |
| Gifts | Touching or having sexual intimacy |
| Invitations to social events | Engaging in multiple roles |
| Entering a personal space without a clear invitation | Extending supervisory time |
| | Meeting outside the supervisory location |
| Exploring content that has unclear relevance to the supervisory or mentorship content | Engaging in psychotherapy within the supervisory context |
| Engaging in sexual or other discriminatory harassment | |

concerning given the significant frequency of occurrence and their potential for exploitation or harm. Such behaviors included showing favoritism based on a personal relationship with a trainee (32%), making a trainee uncomfortable by invading personal space (31%), dating another trainee in the program (26%), making a trainee uncomfortable by asking details of their private life (24%), touching a trainee inappropriately (12%), using a trainee in research/writing without giving appropriate recognition (10%), failing to enforce rules or boundaries out of sympathy for a trainee (9%), asking a trainee on a date (8%), and asking a trainee to lie for the supervisor (5%). Although some of these behaviors do not qualify as misconduct, they all represent behaviors that could be considered on the "slippery slope."

Ellis et al. (2014) surveyed clinical trainees from multiple non–M.D. mental health disciplines about inadequate and harmful supervision. *Harmful supervision* was defined as supervisory actions that failed to put the trainee's best interests above those of the supervisor. In their study, 35% of trainees reported receiving harmful supervision at the time of the study and 51% reported having received harmful supervision at some point in their training. It was also noted that harmful supervision events were not isolated (Ellis et al. 2014). This study not only solicited self-report responses of harmful supervision but also asked participants to respond to empirically derived, specific criteria of harmful behaviors. Respondents noted a much greater number of incidences when responding to inquiries about specific criteria. More than 20% of trainees may have unknowingly received harmful supervision because they may have been unaware of what *constitutes* harmful clinical supervision. Furthermore, 63% of trainees did not report self-identified harmful supervision (Ellis et al. 2014).

It remains unclear what factors drive harmful supervision. The inherent power differential and expectations embedded in the supervisory relationship may place trainees at risk given that supervisors are generally perceived as trustworthy despite having an evaluative role and trainees are expected to divulge information without reciprocation. Psychodynamic psychotherapy supervision, with its integral process of exploring countertransference, may place residents in an even more vulnerable position by virtue of the expectation that they share more personal information. Supervisors must clearly understand the difference between supervision and psychotherapy and avoid engaging in the latter with trainees (Frawley-O'Dea and Sarnat 2001). Any material that relates to work with a patient is part of supervision. A trainee's personal life and problems unrelated to this material, however, are not. Without careful monitoring, supervisors may be at risk of exploring personal factors that go beyond the scope or clinical relevance to the patient at hand. Even if personal disclosures are relevant to the clinical material, supervisors must be mindful of their impact on the resident; if such disclosures are destabilizing, the supervisor must limit discussions or explore the option of personal psychotherapy for the resident if the resident is not already in therapy. When personal dynamics are present that interfere with the treatment of patients and are not easily resolved, a recommendation to psychotherapy is warranted (Gold 2004).

Multiple relationships in supervision may also place supervisors at risk of boundary transgressions, such as when a supervisor has an additional relationship(s) with a resident beyond the supervisory relationship. Multiple relationships become problematic when "(a) there is a power differential between the two parties and (b) the multiple roles they have in relationship with one another put the person with less power at risk for exploitation or harm" (Bernard and Goodyear 2019, p. 259). Depending on the training context, multiple relationships may be common and not necessarily problematic (Gottlieb et al. 2007); examples include a supervisor inviting a trainee to join a professional committee that they chair, coauthor a manuscript, or engage in a research project for which the supervisor is a principal investigator. These relationships are not necessarily forbidden but warrant careful monitoring for exploitation.

Supervisors must identify and be mindful of potential boundary concerns within the supervisory relationship. Reflecting on personal attributes that may put them at risk can be helpful. For example, a supervisor whose personality is expressive and encourages openness may conflict with a particular resident's sense of interpersonal space or willingness to divulge personal information. Without forethought, such a supervisor may make the resident uncomfortable. It is important to consider one's role and how this role is performed with residents. One might also review organizational codes of ethics for guidance. Regrettably, unlike the American Psychological Association Ethics Code (American Psychological Association 2017), the American Psychiatric Association does not address ethical issues related to supervision (American Psychiatric Association 2013). Furthermore, setting the framework of supervision, as previously suggested, may include clarifying what material is generally shared within the supervisory context and how the supervisor intends to avoid slipping into the psychotherapist role.

Intentional boundary crossings should be made with sensitivity to individual differences, as with boundaries within a clinical setting. Each potential crossing should be reviewed on its own merit, considering the supervisor's intent and motive and the resident's particular situation and background, including cultural and ethical considerations, and in the context of community norms, ethical codes, and legal standards. To prevent an inadvertent crossing or violation, it is incumbent upon the supervisor to self-reflect. As with potential boundary encroachments within psychotherapy, supervisors might consider whether a the potential behavior will lead to a possible boundary transgression by asking the following (Barnett and Molzon 2014; Burian and Slimp 2000; Pope and Keith-Spiegel 2008):

1. What are the potential best and worst outcomes from either crossing or not crossing the boundary?
2. Will engaging in the behavior be in the resident's best interest?
3. Will acting in this way be consistent with the supervisor's obligations to the resident?
4. Does the supervisor have any uneasy feelings, doubts, and confusions? (If so, explore what's causing them and their implications.)
5. Will this action possibly result in harm to the resident?
6. What might be the impact on other, uninvolved residents or staff should a given behavior be acted on?
7. What are the literature and ethics codes for supervision?
8. What might be the professional and personal benefit to *both* the supervisor and the resident?

Supervisors might also consider consulting trusted colleagues to provide added perspectives and to help expose any blind spots or biases. If the supervisor decides to cross a boundary, that supervisor must be continually vigilant to safeguard against any change in resident or supervisor perspective or to identify evidence of discomfort or harm.

If a supervisor has concerns about an ongoing inadvertent boundary crossing or violation, the following considerations may help clarify the situation (Walker and Clark 1999):

1. Are there any strong feelings toward a resident that may lead to conflating personal and professional caring?
2. Have supervisory sessions been extended?
3. Have any inappropriate communications or diversions from normal supervisory behaviors occurred?
4. Is there a desire to make off-hour telephone calls to and from your resident or to give gifts?
5. Are you overprotecting and overidentifying with the resident?
6. Are you engaging in more self-disclosures than usual?
7. Are you touching or comforting the resident or desiring or having sexual contact?

Repairing a supervisory relationship that has been ruptured by a boundary encroachment may be challenging but is essential. At times, crossings may not be obvious to a supervisor unless the trainee points them out. The resident may withdraw from the supervisory relationship, ask fewer questions, engage less in discussions, or simply appear less involved. If such behavior changes occur, the supervisor should reflect carefully. If a boundary transgression is of concern, the supervisor must reflect on how the transgression developed and the options for resolution. Particularly in the case of a boundary violation, it may be important to consult the professional code of ethics and, where necessary, a trusted colleague or risk manager for the institution. Once options for managing the transgression have been considered, and depending on risk management advice and the scope of the transgression, it will be important for the supervisor to initiate an honest and open discussion with the resident. Start by respectfully acknowledging the situation and the concern for any impact it may have had. Depending on the situation, it may be helpful to advise the resident to seek consultation from a trusted peer or supervisor and to inform the resident that you are also seeking consultation. This approach may help diffuse any tension or confusion (Gutheil and Gabbard 1993; Walker and Clark 1999; Watkins 2019).

Should a resident confront the supervisor about a boundary crossing or violation, it may be difficult for that supervisor to maintain a stance of openness and nondefensiveness (Watkins 2019). It is important to be self-reflective and open to examining one's own behavior while respectfully recognizing the reality of the rupture as described by the resident.

Working with the resident to process the event and to find an appropriate and satisfactory resolution of the situation while prioritizing the supervisory relationship is critical. The hope is a return to a healthy and functioning supervisory alliance, if appropriate. If the transgression is significant, outside counsel may be required and training leadership may need to be informed (Watkins 2019).

Maintaining good interpersonal boundaries in clinical supervision is clearly important, just as it is in psychotherapy. It is the key responsibility of the supervisor to guard against violations and to reflect deeply on any intent to cross a boundary. Finally, supervisors should seek training, if available, to increase awareness of potential boundary crossings and violations, with the hope of reducing inappropriate, inadvertent, and often harmful behaviors.

## CONCLUSION

Thoughtful attention to the learning goals and relational aspects of supervision is critical to success. Supervisors are educators and role models of substantial importance. Monitoring the relationship for boundary crossings and incorporating aspects of mentorship further enhance supervision.

### — KEY POINTS —

- Supervision must have defined learning goals and clear contractual obligations for each party.
- Mentorship is a highly valued and important part of trainee supervision but lacks complete confidentiality based on the supervisor's role as evaluator.
- Maintaining boundaries within supervision is critical and a fundamental responsibility of the supervisor.
- Intentional boundary crossings should be made with sensitivity to individual differences and *always* with the best interests of the trainee in mind.
- Ideally, supervisors should seek training to increase awareness of potential boundary crossings and violations, with the hope of reducing inappropriate, inadvertent, and often harmful behaviors that impact not only the trainee but also the educational environment.

# REFERENCES


American Psychiatric Association: The Principles of Medical Ethics With Annotations Especially Applicable to Psychiatry. Arlington, VA, American Psychiatric Association, 2013. Available at: https://www.psychiatry.org/psychiatrists/practice/ethics. Accessed October 1, 2019.

American Psychological Association: Ethical Principles of Psychologists and Code of Conduct, Including 2010 and 2016 Amendments. Washington, DC, American Psychological Association, 2017. Available at: http://www.apa.org/ethics. Accessed October 1, 2019.

Association for Counselor Education and Supervision: Appendix D: Task Force report: best practice in clinical supervision, January 18, 2011, in Using Technology to Enhance Clinical Supervision. Edited by Rousmaniere T, Renfro-Michel E. Alexandria, VA, American Counseling Association, 2016, pp 285–302

Barnett JE: Ethical issues in clinical supervision. Clin Psychol 64:14–20, 2011

Barnett JE, Molzon CH: Clinical supervision of psychotherapy: essential ethics issues for supervisors and supervisees. J Clin Psychol 70(11):1051–1061, 2014

Bennett-Levy J, Lee N, Travers K, et al: Cognitive therapy from the inside: enhancing therapist skills through practicing what we preach. Behav Cogn Psychother 31:145–163, 2003

Bernard JM, Goodyear RK: Fundamentals of Clinical Supervision, 6th Edition. Upper Saddle River, NJ, Merrill, 2019

Burian BK, Slimp AOC: Social dual-role relationships during internship: a decision-making model. Prof Psychol Res Pract 31(3):332–338, 2000

Clark RA, Harden SL, Johnson WB: Mentor relationships in clinical psychology doctoral training: results of a national survey. Teach Psychol 27:262–268, 2000

Dorsey S, Kerns S, Lucid L, et al: Objective coding of content and techniques in workplace-based supervision of an EBT in public mental health. Implementation Sci 13(1):19, 2018

Ellis MV, Berger L, Hanus AE, et al: Inadequate and harmful clinical supervision: testing a revised framework and assessing occurrence. Couns Psychol 42(4):434–472, 2014

Falender CA, Shafranske EP: Clinical Supervision: A Competency-Based Approach. Washington, DC, American Psychological Association, 2004

Feldman MD, Arean PA, Marshall SJ, et al: Does mentoring matter? Results from a survey of faculty mentees at a large health sciences university. Med Educ Online 15, 2010

Frawley O'Dea MG, Sarnat JE: The Supervisory Relationship: A Contemporary Psychodynamic Approach. New York, Guilford, 2001

Fulton J: Mentorship: excellence in the mundane. British Journal of Healthcare Assistants 7(3):142–144, 2013

Gold JH: Reflections on psychodynamic psychotherapy supervision for psychiatrists in clinical practice. J Psychiatr Pract 10(3):162–169, 2004

Gottlieb MC, Robinson K, Younggren JN: Multiple relations in supervision: guidance for administrators, supervisors, and students. Prof Psychol Res Pract 38:241–247, 2007

Gutheil TG, Gabbard GO: The concept of boundaries in clinical practice: theoretical and risk-management dimensions. Am J Psychiatry 150:188–196, 1993

Harms S, Bogie BJM, Lizius A, et al: From good to great: learners' perceptions of the qualities of effective medical teachers and clinical supervisors in psychiatry. Can Med Educ J 10(3):e17–e26, 2019

Jackson VA, Palepu A, Szalacha L, et al: "Having the right chemistry:" a qualitative study of mentoring in academic medicine. Acad Med 78:328–334, 2003

Johnson WB: Transformational supervision: when supervisors mentor. Prof Psychol Res Pract 38:259–267, 2007

Kaslow NJ, Mascaro NA: Mentoring interns and postdoctoral residents in academic health sciences center. J Clin Psychol Med Settings 14:191–196, 2007

Kilgallon K, Thompson J: Mentoring in Nursing and Healthcare: A Practical Approach. Chichester, UK, Wiley-Blackwell, 2012

Koopman RJ, Thiedke CC: Views of family medicine department chairs about mentoring junior faculty. Med Teach 27:734–737, 2005

Ladany N: Psychotherapy supervision: what lies beneath. Psychother Res 14:1–19, 2004

Laschober TC, Turner de Tormes L, Kinkade K: Mentoring support from clinical supervisors: mentor motives and associations to counselor work-to-nonwork conflict. J Subst Abuse Treat 44:186–192, 2013

Mehr KE, Ladany N, Caskie GIL: Trainee nondisclosure in supervision: what are they not telling you? Couns Psychother Res 10(2):103–113, 2010

Milne DL, Reiser RP: A Manual for Evidence-Based Supervision. Hoboken, NJ, John Wiley and Sons, 2017

Nelson ML, Friedlander ML: A close look at conflictual supervisory relationships: the trainee's perspective. J Couns Psychol 48(4):384–395, 2001

Newman M, Ravindranath D, Figueroa S, Jibson MD: Perceptions of supervision in an outpatient psychiatry clinic. Acad Psychiatry 40:153–156, 2016

Pope KS, Keith-Spiegel P: A practical approach to boundaries in psychotherapy: making decisions, bypassing blunders, and mending fences. J Clin Psychol 64(5):638–652, 2008

Recupero PR, Cooney MC, Rayner C, et al: Supervisor-trainee relationship boundaries in medical education. Med Teach 27(6):484–488, 2005

Sambunjak D, Straus S, Marušik A: Mentoring in academic medicine: a systematic review. JAMA 296:1103–1115, 2006

Shanfield SB, Mohl PC, Matthews KL, Hetherly V: Quantitative assessment of the behavior of psychotherapy supervisors. Am J Psychiatry 149(3):352–357, 1992

Singh A, Chun KYS: "From the margins to the center": moving towards a resilience-based model of supervision for queer people of color supervisors. Train Educ Prof Psychol 4(1):36–46, 2010

Stenfors-Hayes T, Hult H, Dahlgren LO: What does it mean to be a good teacher and clinical supervisor in medical education? Adv Health Sci Educ Theory Pract 16(2):197–210, 2011

Straus SE, Chatur F, Taylor M: Issues in the mentor-mentee relationship in academic medicine: qualitative study. Acad Med 84:135–139, 2009

Vasquez MJT: Psychologist as clinical supervisor: promoting ethical practice. Prof Psychol Res Pract 23:196–202, 1992

Walker R, Clark JJ: Heading off boundary problems: clinical supervision as risk management. Psychiatr Serv 50(11):1435–1439, 1999

Watkins CE: Ruptures in the supervisory alliance, in Supervision in Psychiatric Practice: Practical Approaches Across Venues and Providers. Edited by De Golia SG, Corcoran KM. Washington, DC, American Psychiatric Association Publishing, 2019

Williams LL, Levine JB, Malhotra S, Holtzheimer P: The good-enough mentoring relationship. Acad Psychiatry 8:111–115, 2004

## CHAPTER 5

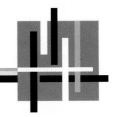

# TAKING A SCHOLARLY APPROACH TO PSYCHIATRIC EDUCATION

Laurel J. Bessey, M.D.
Art Walaszek, M.D.

**Medical** education can feel very reactive. Educators must address personnel crises, respond to the latest regulations, manage reductions in resources, and resolve many other problems. We of course *should* (and in some cases *must*) respond in a timely, thoughtful, and thorough way to the changing needs of our learners, our faculty, and ultimately our patients. Without a framework that supports efforts to improve psychiatric education, faculty may feel frustrated, overwhelmed, and ultimately burned out by concurrent clinical and educational demands: putting out fires rather than cultivating a forest that is less vulnerable to fire.

We believe a *scholarly approach* provides psychiatric educators with just such a framework. A psychiatric educator could employ a scholarly approach to any of these educational tasks: creating and giving lectures; facilitating small-group discussions; supervising, mentoring, or other advising; developing curricula or instructional methods; and administering the educational program (Fincher et al. 2000). More specifically, any education leader can take the following steps (Fincher et al. 2000):

1. Develop vision and mission statements, goals, and objectives that are clear, realistic, and measurable and are consistent with departmental and organizational goals.
2. Apply relevant concepts in the educational literature to local projects and assemble the resources needed to develop and implement a plan.
3. Use methods consistent with the intended outcome and identify and address potential barriers to implementation.
4. Measure outcomes and determine whether desired changes and results were achieved.
5. Share results—both process and content—with others, including local stakeholders (e.g., learners, faculty) and educators outside of the institution.
6. Actively seek feedback, respond to critiques, and glean lessons for future projects.

A scholarly approach also serves as the foundation for *educational scholarship*, which advances knowledge in psychiatric education through peer review and publication (Simpson et al. 2013). Faced with an educational task or problem, the psychiatric educator may ask the following questions:

- *What exactly is the problem we are trying to solve?* The first step is clearly defining the problem. Is it an educational problem—that is, a problem that an educational intervention could address? Systems or personnel problems require different solutions.
- *What does the medical education literature say about how to solve this particular problem?* If prior educational scholarship has already produced a solution, the educator should consider that solution rather than create something new. On the other hand, even if a solution is already available, perhaps local circumstances warrant a scholarly project.
- *Is this an opportunity to contribute to the medical education literature?* Will the outcome (e.g., dissemination of knowledge, promotion of scholarly activity, career development) justify the effort (e.g., faculty time, money, other resources, opportunity cost)?

Attitudes most likely to benefit a psychiatric educator using a scholarly approach include curiosity, lack of judgment, openness to change, and appreciation of the backgrounds and values of their learners and colleagues. Adopting a scholarly approach requires the ability to identify educational resources, including current educational scholarship—a topic we cover in the next section. Later in the chapter we highlight a specific critical task of psychiatric educators—designing and implementing a curriculum—as particularly well suited for a scholarly approach. Finally, we discuss educational research and disseminating the results of educational projects.

## FINDING RESOURCES TO SUPPORT A SCHOLARLY APPROACH

Topics in medical education, such as curriculum design, are rarely covered in medical school and residency. Aspiring psychiatric educators may need education in this area. Seminal articles in medical education exist, several of which we cite in this chapter; for a compilation, see Sullivan (2015). Our preferred reference for curriculum design is *Curriculum Development for Medical Education: A Six-Step Approach* (Thomas et al. 2016), which we cover in greater detail herein. The Best Evidence in Medical Education Collaboration, sponsored by the Association for Medical Education in Europe (AMEE), publishes systematic reviews of educational topics; these are handy for educators looking for a summary of the evidence regarding a specific educational strategy (Best Evidence in Medical Education Collaboration 2019).

We recommend that all psychiatric educators regularly read *Academic Psychiatry*, the primary journal of psychiatric education (2018 impact factor [IF] 1.880). Other noteworthy journals include *Academic Medicine* (IF 5.083), *Medical Teacher* (IF 2.706), *Teaching and Learning in Medicine* (IF 2.216), *BMC Medical Education* (IF 1.870), and the *Journal of Graduate Medical Education* (IF not reported). A well-constructed PubMed search may help psychiatric educators find many articles relevant to their project (for a review of search strategies in the medical education literature, see Haig and Dozier 2003). Familiarity with these journals will also help educators determine the types of articles likely to be published, which is of benefit if one plans to disseminate the outcome of projects. Becoming a manuscript reviewer to gain further insights into effective dissemination is also helpful (for guidelines, see Roberts et al. 2004).

Local educational resources within a medical school, such as seminars, workshops, webinars, longitudinal programs, or other curricula meant for medical educators, are valuable and offer opportunities for networking and collaboration across departments. An assistant or associate dean for faculty development (or someone with a comparable title) may help you learn about local resources and opportunities, including grants to support educational scholarship. A medical librarian is often an invaluable resource for conducting an effective literature search. Joining your medical school or university teaching academy (or similar organization) can connect you with the wider community of educators at your institution. Your medical school or university information technology department may offer resources to help faculty with the development and implementation of curricula.

Professional medical associations are significant resources for faculty members seeking guidance or mentorship. Organizations most involved in psychiatric education include the Association for Academic Psychiatry (AAP; www.academicpsychiatry.org), Association of Directors of Medical Student Education in Psychiatry (ADMSEP; www.admsep.org), and American Association of Directors of Psychiatric Residency Training (AADPRT; www.aadprt.org). These organizations, along with the American Association of Chairs of Departments of Psychiatry, belong to a consortium that oversees the journal *Academic Psychiatry*; members of one or more of these organizations can receive copies of the journal.

- AAP focuses on career development and the dissemination of best practices in psychiatric education. Its annual meeting provides opportunities for learning educational techniques (via workshops and plenaries as well as their Master Educator series), networking with colleagues and identifying mentors, and dissemination (by presenting at workshops). Educational activities at the AAP annual meeting tend to be interactive and built on adult learning principles. AAP also grants awards to residents and junior faculty who demonstrate promise as educators.
- ADMSEP is an organization of psychiatric educators who participate in medical student education in psychiatry and behavioral sciences. Its annual meeting includes workshops on educational content and methods and is meant to promote networking and collegial support.
- AADPRT promotes the education of psychiatry residents and fellows through the education and support of residency training directors, fellowship directors, and faculty and staff involved in graduate medical education (GME). AADPRT has a very active email listserv that fosters communication and supports education between annual meetings. Annual meetings include a pre-meeting, various plenaries and educational workshops, and a parallel meeting for program administrators.

The American Psychiatric Association offers rich educational content. Subspecialty societies, as described in Chapter 14, have active educational components. Organizations outside of psychiatry that may be of interest include the Accreditation Council for Graduate Medical Education (ACGME; www.acgme.org), which hosts an annual educational conference as well as courses and workshops for faculty involved in

GME, produces the *Journal of Graduate Medical Education*, and aggregates resources for program directors on its website; the AMEE, which oversees the journal *Medical Teacher*; and the Association of American Medical Colleges (AAMC; www.aamc.org), which offers professional development courses and "affinity groups" such as the Group on Educational Affairs. The Accreditation Council on Continuing Medical Education (www.accme.org), American Board of Psychiatry and Neurology (ABPN; www.abpn.com), and Liaison Committee on Medical Education (LCME; www.lcme.org) may serve as valuable resources for psychiatric educators. For example, the ABPN offers grants to support innovative educational efforts in a variety of areas, not just related to board certification. Psychiatric educators also may benefit from a host of web-based resources; please see Table 5–1.

Personal and environmental resources are necessary to adopt a scholarly approach. A "personal infrastructure," including negotiating for protected time for educational work, thinking strategically (e.g., keeping in mind long-term educational goals), planning prospectively, and adopting a specific timeline, is critical (Sullivan 2018). Educational projects are more likely to be effective when an educator collaborates with others; joining educational organizations and attending their annual meetings may lead to such relationships, and participating in social media (e.g., Twitter hashtag #MedEd) may also lead to partnerships (Sullivan 2018). An even more powerful approach would be to develop or join a medical education practice-based research network (see "Designing an Educational Research Project") (Schwartz et al. 2016). Senior educators can "pass it on" by mentoring or sponsoring junior faculty or may develop a local community of education scholars and promote the educational skills of their colleagues (Sullivan 2018).

## DESIGNING AND IMPLEMENTING A CURRICULUM

One particular educational task well suited to a scholarly approach is *curriculum design*. Both the LCME and ACGME require curricula with clearly defined goals and objectives and with which learner outcomes are identified and measured. These requirements at both the undergraduate medical education (UME) and GME levels are evaluated through a rigorous self-study process and associated site visits (Accreditation Council for Graduate Medical Education 2019; Liaison Committee on Medical Education 2019).

What exactly is a curriculum? We define *curriculum* as the aggregate of planned educational experiences associated with a particular topic, course,

**Table 5–1.** Web-based resources for psychiatric educators

| Organization | Website | Description |
|---|---|---|
| MedEdPortal | www.mededportal.org | Repository of peer-reviewed educational materials may help identify already available materials |
| Association of Directors of Medical Student Education in Psychiatry (ADMSEP) | www.admsep.org/csi-emodules.php?c=emodules-description | 14 Web-based educational modules intended for use with medical students as part of ADMSEP's Clinical Simulation Initiative |
| National Neuroscience Curriculum Initiative (NNCI) | www.nncionline.org | Free resources to support teaching residents about the neurobiological underpinnings of psychiatry; funded by National Institute of Mental Health |
| American Association of Directors of Psychiatric Residency Training (AADPRT) Virtual Training Office | www.aadprt.org | Many educational resources, including curricula that AADPRT's Curriculum Committee has vetted (AADPRT membership required) |
| *Journal of Graduate Medical Education* | www.jgme.org/page/ripouts | Includes "rip outs," which are brief summaries of specific educational topics |
| Portal of Geriatrics Online Education (POGOe) | www.pogoe.org | Curricula specific to geriatrics, including geriatric psychiatry |
| Academy of Consultation-Liaison Psychiatry (ACLP) | www.clpsychiatry.org/member-resources/resident-curriculum/ | Consultation-liaison curriculum for psychiatry residents |
| Association for Medical Education in Europe (AMEE)'s *MedEdPublish* | www.mededpublish.org | Open-access journal of articles about medical education with postpublication peer review (i.e., articles are published first, then peer reviewed, then revised if necessary) |

or program. This section describes a systematic process for designing, implementing, and assessing a curriculum. We also discuss curriculum development as a potential opportunity for research. For a deeper dive, we recommend *Curriculum Development for Medical Education: A Six-Step Approach* (Thomas et al. 2016). Here we summarize that approach.

## Conducting a Needs Assessment

The first step in developing a curriculum is a *needs assessment*. A new curriculum may be needed because of a gap in addressing a health care problem or because of new regulatory requirements. After identifying the topic, examine what is currently being done to address it, including by patients, learners, health care providers, the health care system, and the community. Consider the ideal approach to the topic and how this differs from what is occurring. Differences provide potential target areas for the curriculum.

After identifying the problem or gap to be addressed, determine the audience for the curriculum. The UME or GME audience will generally be psychiatry residents, medical students, and faculty. Outside of these settings, the curriculum may involve teaching other groups, such as patients, community members, law enforcement, and other health care professionals. We focus here on curriculum development for residents, fellows, and medical students. The faculty teaching a new curriculum may have educational needs themselves, such as learning new educational methods. In determining need, educators should take into account other considerations about learners, teaching faculty, and the teaching environment as outlined in Table 5–2 and determine the needs of stakeholders, such as accrediting bodies, program directors, course or clerkship directors, and others.

## Gathering Information

Completing a needs assessment requires information. A review of the literature is essential and may provide current best practices, evidence-based reviews, original studies, textbooks, and curricula used by other institutions. Educators may gather more information about local circumstances by, for example, holding a focus group, deploying a survey, reviewing current outcomes (e.g., scores on examinations or patient satisfaction surveys), and identifying relevant departmental or institutional policies and procedures. We distinguish content expertise (what will be taught) from expertise in educational methods (*how* it will be taught—primarily the subject of this chapter). Educators who are not content experts themselves may need to consult content experts.

**Table 5–2.** Information for needs assessment

| | |
|---|---|
| **Learners and teaching faculty** | |
| | Who they are |
| | Current knowledge and skill level |
| | Previous experiences and training related to topic |
| | Learning/Teaching style, preferences, and needs |
| | Learning/Teaching ability |
| | Attitudes related to the topic |
| | Available resources |
| **Teaching environment** | |
| | Related curricula and faculty development |
| | Teaching setting (e.g., lecture, small group, clinical supervision) |
| | Facilities |
| | Available time |
| | Cost of curriculum and available funding |
| | Support staff |
| | Other needed resources |

Comparing the current curriculum, outcomes, and environment with state-of-the-art educational practices will identify gaps and inform the needs assessment—and may help educators determine if they should adapt a previously developed curriculum or create a new one.

## Writing Goals and Objectives

The next step is to use the information gathered in the needs assessment and literature review to write clear *goals and objectives* for the curriculum. Goals and objectives guide the creation of curriculum content, may suggest instructional strategies, communicate what the curriculum seeks to accomplish, and may help determine methods to assess learner outcomes and evaluate the curriculum. Goals communicate to learners and other stakeholders the purpose of the curriculum and the intended outcomes. Goals tend to be broad, require a longer time frame, include final results and outcomes, and may not be measurable. Goals are often based on the curriculum as a whole. Learning objectives are more specific and measurable, occur in a shorter time frame, and often include how the learner will achieve the goals. Multiple sets of learning objectives generally exist in each curriculum that arise from individual didactic or other planned learning experiences. The remainder of this section focuses on the process of writing effective learning objectives.

Specific and measurable learning objectives usually answer the question "Who will do how much, how well, of what, by when?" (Thomas et al. 2016). Learning objectives should include a verb, a noun, and adjectives that answer this question. Different types and levels of learning objectives exist, including learner, process, and outcome-driven. Learning objectives may also be specific to a person or to a program. The educator uses the needs assessment to write learner-based objectives, which fall into three categories:

- *Knowledge* objectives may involve various cognitive processes based on a revision of Bloom's taxonomy (Anderson et al. 2001). These processes, in increasing order of complexity, include remembering (factual knowledge), understanding, applying, analyzing, evaluating, and creating; levels may not develop in this order (Anderson et al. 2001).
- *Skills* objectives include psychomotor tasks, behaviors, or performance-based activities that can often be observed in a clinical or simulated setting.
- *Attitudinal* objectives focus on developing or changing specific values, beliefs, and emotions and may emphasize importance or appreciation of the learning material.

GME and UME require competency-based education models. Learning objectives should be based on competencies, subcompetencies, and milestones as defined by the ACGME and AAMC (Association of American Medical Colleges 2019; Englander et al. 2013; Psychiatry Milestone Group 2015). Educators should also consider institution- and program-specific missions, objectives, milestones, and goals. Certain competencies may be more likely to include particular types of objectives (i.e., assessing competency in medical knowledge requires writing knowledge objectives). Mapping goals and objectives to competencies may also inform future curriculum development.

Content experts, educational methodology experts, learners, and other stakeholders should review and comment on draft goals and objectives to ensure they are written clearly and comprehensively enough to address the identified needs and requirements of the curriculum.

## Selecting an Instructional Method

It is important to select *instructional methods* to aid in achieving the curriculum's goals and objectives. Using multiple educational approaches enhances learners' engagement and ability to attain competence. Adult learners are independent, self-directed, and internally motivated. They have lived experience that is useful for future learning, and value learning that helps solve their real-world problems (Kaufman 2003). Resources, including time, faculty preferences, teaching environment, and financial support, may also influence which instructional methods are used. See Chapter 1 for more background regarding principles of adult learning.

Table 5–3 lists several instructional methods that may be appropriate for each category of learner-based objective. One method may serve to achieve multiple objectives, and a combination of multiple methods (e.g., reading followed by discussion) may achieve one objective. Some methods are self-directed by learners, whereas others are directed by faculty; a mix of both may help promote lifelong learning, an important competency for physicians.

## Implementing the Curriculum

Ideally, in a culture of continuous quality improvement, implementing and assessing the curriculum should go hand-in-hand so educators can regularly fine-tune it. A strategic approach includes engaging and gaining support from stakeholders and anticipating and addressing barriers to implementation. Stakeholders include learners, faculty involved in deploying the curriculum, accrediting bodies, and many others. Table 5–4 lists stakeholders to consider engaging and why they are important. Involving stakeholders in earlier steps (e.g., needs assessment) helps with engagement and with identifying both barriers and solutions to implementation.

**Table 5–3.** Instructional methods for learning objectives

| Knowledge objectives | Skills objectives | Attitudinal objectives |
|---|---|---|
| Reading | Standardized patients | Reading |
| Lecture | Simulations | Discussion |
| Peer teaching | Demonstration | Experience |
| Online modules | Roleplay | Reflective writing |
| Discussion | Supervised clinical experience | Role models |
| Problem-based learning | Review video or audio of skills | Roleplay |
| Team-based learning | | |
| Flipped classroom | | |

**Table 5–4.** Stakeholders in medical education

| Stakeholder | Importance |
|---|---|
| Learners | Need to see how the curriculum supports their goals<br>Will be participating in activities |
| Faculty | Needed to teach the curriculum<br>Need to feel that the methods, goals, and objectives are worth their time<br>Enthusiasm will likely improve overall reception of the course |
| Leaders and administrators* | Provide resources (e.g., funding, space, time)<br>Can help gain faculty support for the curriculum (providing financial support or enthusiasm)<br>Need to address concerns in order to gain resources and support<br>Determine how the curriculum will further institutional goals and values |
| Professional societies | Potential source of funding<br>May have important guidelines or requirements that can help garner support from other stakeholders<br>Can provide opportunities for faculty development |
| Accrediting bodies | Provide accreditation for the institution |

*Dean, department chair, program or course director, departmental or medical school administrator, medical education staff (e.g., residency coordinator).

Next, identify available resources and then request more resources to either implement or modify the curriculum to fit those available. Such resources include funding, facilities, faculty, patients, simulators, standardized patients, and support staff. Support from stakeholders may lead to an increase in resources, such as hiring staff or conducting faculty development.

Faculty may need to build skills and knowledge to successfully implement the curriculum, which will require an investment of their time and energy, often the most challenging limiting factors. Faculty development could consist of communication (e.g., email, newsletter, faculty meetings), a curriculum specifically for faculty ("train the trainer"), or having faculty train through professional medical associations. Providing continuing medical education credit may encourage faculty to attend development activities.

To determine if a curriculum is effective and if learners are achieving the desired objectives, educators must adopt preexisting assessments or develop and implement new ones. All stakeholders should be aware of the assessment process from the outset (see section "Assessing Outcomes" later). The next step is introducing the curriculum. One approach is to start with a pilot phase, which allows for gathering feedback from participants and modifying the curriculum prior to its full implementation. Another approach is to introduce the curriculum in multiple phases, which can be helpful when a change in the clinical learning environment or local educational culture is necessary. Introducing the curricular components slowly allows for a shift in the educational culture, and evaluation allows for revision. If the need for a new curriculum is urgent, full implementation may need to come first, followed by outcomes assessment and curriculum modification.

## Promoting Inclusion and Cultural Competence

Developing a curriculum that is inclusive of and sensitive to the needs of all learners and faculty members helps ensure that the curriculum is effective and durable. Learners and faculty members bring to the educational setting various cultural backgrounds and personal experiences. Cultural humility, cultural competence, structural competence, health care disparities, and inclusive teaching are in and of themselves critical topics for students, residents, fellows, and faculty members.

Psychiatrists care for an increasingly diverse patient population, and regulatory bodies such as the LCME and ACGME are placing greater emphasis on diversity, equity, and inclusion. We recommend that all educators consider their curricula through this lens, including explicitly addressing the cultural components within them. Educational outcomes of cultural competency curricula using a variety of teaching strategies, including immersion, simulation, discussion groups, lectures, reflection, educational technology, case-based learning, writing essays, presentations, readings, and videos—ranging from 20 minutes of intervention to 600 hours of training embedded throughout a curriculum—have been mixed (Brottman et al. 2020). Training the faculty delivering the curriculum, selecting a model to guide it, using a blend of educational approaches, and acknowledging the lifelong nature of learning to provide culturally competent health care may improve effectiveness (Brottman et al. 2020). We recommend incorporating cultural competency as a thread throughout multiple curricula. The Cultural Formulation Interview included in DSM-5 (American Psychiatric Association 2013) can be a valuable resource in teaching medical students and residents about psychiatric diagnosis and treatment. We also recommend *Sociocultural Issues in Psychiatry: A Casebook and Curriculum* (Trinh and Chen 2019) as a resource. Further discussion of diversity and inclusion may be found in Chapter 6.

## Assessing Outcomes

Educators assess the quality of a curriculum by measuring two sets of outcomes: to what extent learners achieved the educational objectives and to what extent the curriculum itself was effective.

### *ASSESSING THE LEARNER*

Assessment of a learner can provide information about both individual learner performance and the success of the curriculum in attaining learning objectives. Clarify at the start of the curriculum the assessments to be used, how they relate to the overarching goals (e.g., graduating medical school), and the expectations for learners. Assessment of learners falls into two categories that differ in their purpose.

- *Formative assessment* offers learners low-stakes opportunities to receive feedback and identify areas for improvement or further study.
- *Summative assessment* focuses on overall performance, asks high-stakes questions (e.g., did this student pass or fail?), and allows judgment about a learner's grade, certification, entrustment of a professional activity, promotion, or graduation.

In competency-based medical education, different types of assessment may be mapped to milestones or other summative descriptions of performance. This allows directors of courses or entire programs to view the specific curriculum within the context of the overall curricula, with a view to identifying gaps and areas for improvement. Further discussion of assessment strategies is available in Chapter 10.

### *ASSESSING THE CURRICULUM*

Educators should assess the curriculum as a whole to foster continuous quality improvement. Examining aggregate learner outcomes, evaluating learners' performance on standardized examinations (e.g., National Board of Medical Examiners subject examinations, the Psychiatry Resident-In-Training Examination, or the ABPN initial certification), and soliciting and reviewing learners' feedback allow an evaluation of the entire curriculum. A curriculum developer may periodically review relevant literature to see if the curriculum meets the latest educational developments and standards. The categories of formative and summative assessment also apply to curriculum assessment (Table 5–5).

A curriculum has a natural lifespan. Educators should assess their curriculum with a view to enhancing, maintaining, and, eventually, ending it. Educators may need to change the content, instructional methods, assessment, training of faculty, or faculty themselves. Ongoing assessment may identify a need for new resources or to modify the curriculum to match changing resources. Changes in the accreditation requirements, advances in the psychiatric knowledge base, updates in psychiatric practice, and changes in the clinical learning environment may require a revision of the curriculum or a new curriculum, and the cycle of design may begin again.

**Table 5–5.** Modes of formative and summative feedback in medical education

| Formative | Summative |
|---|---|
| **Learner** | Midterm or final examination |
| Pretest | National examinations (i.e., U.S. Medical Licensing Examination, Psychiatry Resident-In-Training Examination, American Board of Psychiatry and Neurology boards) |
| Quizzes | |
| Reflection or other writing assignments | |
| Formal and informal feedback on practice performance | Objective structured clinical examination (observed structured clinical encounters or clinical skills evaluation/verification) |
| Self-assessment questionnaire | |
| **Curriculum** | Biannual milestones report by clinical competency committee |
| Course component evaluations during the course | Final clinical evaluation results |
| Informal suggestions | Entrustable Professional Activities rating |
| Learner questions | Aggregate examination results |
| Faculty evaluations | National test pass rates or averages across a program or school |
| Further literature review | National test subscores |
| | Formal course evaluation results |
| | Aggregate pre- vs. posttest comparisons of learners |
| | Course auditing |
| | Faculty evaluations |
| | Accreditation standards |

# PURSUING EDUCATIONAL SCHOLARSHIP

A scholarly approach to developing a curriculum is an opportunity for educational scholarship, advancing knowledge in education through peer review and publication (Simpson et al. 2013). The following discussion provides resources to guide those interested in developing an educational research project. A general resource for medical education is *Research in Medical Education: A Primer for Medical Students* (Association of American Medical Colleges 2015); intended for medical students, this primer has many important considerations and resources for anyone pursuing an educational research project.

## Designing an Educational Research Project

Developing a research project in psychiatry education should involve a systematic process. Beckman and Cook (2007) proposed a three-step process: developing a study question, selecting an appropriate design and methods, and selecting outcomes. Quantitative and qualitative research methods both have merit. Randomized controlled trials, the gold standard for biomedical research, may be less feasible, ethical, and reliable in medical education research. For example, it is often impossible to blind learners to an intervention; education happens in real time, and assigning learners to different educational methods may not be ethical. Strategies to strengthen educational research methods include increasing the sample size (via multiple iterations of the intervention or multiple sites), including a comparison group (a historical control or crossover design or a different site that does not use the intervention), and ensuring standardization via training of teachers (Sullivan 2011b). Alternatively, educational researchers can adopt a qualitative approach or blend a quantitative and qualitative (mixed-method) approach. Qualitative research helps explain why and how something occurs, with collective information from interviews, focus groups, narratives, observations, and document review (Sargeant 2012; Sullivan and Sargeant 2011). To learn more, see Beckman and Cook (2007); Sargeant (2012); Sullivan (2011b); and Sullivan and Sargeant (2011).

Educators must seek institutional review board (IRB) approval or exemption prior to initiating a medical education research project. Educational research about students, residents, and faculty may require IRB approval. Ethical considerations include power differentials between learners and educators, informed consent about involvement, and confidentiality with respect to deidentifying medical education data (Sullivan 2011a). Each institution has a process for IRB approval and exemption

(Dyrbye et al. 2007), so seek guidance from your medical school or sponsoring institution.

Medical education research is a great opportunity for collaboration. GME research, when a residency or fellowship has a limited number of participants, may benefit from collaboration with other institutions to increase sample size and generalizability. Each program must obtain separate IRB approval. One model of collaboration in medical education is a practice-based research network, which creates a framework for educators to work together, pool data, and answer research questions (Schwartz et al. 2016).

Finding funding to support educational research projects is challenging. The quality of published medical education research is associated with the funding for the study (Reed et al. 2007). Educators can identify sources of grant support from professional medical associations and other organizations (e.g., AAMC, AMEE, ABPN) or through their own institutions (e.g., pilot funding from a department or medical school). Other funding sources include foundations (e.g., Arnold P. Gold Foundation, Robert Wood Johnson Foundation, Josiah Macy Jr. Foundation) and federal agencies (e.g., Agency for Healthcare Research and Quality, Centers for Disease Control and Prevention, National Institutes of Health, U.S. Veterans Affairs Department). See Gruppen and Durning (2016) for a comprehensive list.

## Disseminating the Outcome of an Educational Project

Educators may wish to disseminate the outcome of their educational projects in order to share ideas or to promote collaboration with others, fulfill requirements for scholarly activities, and aid in promotion and tenure. Dissemination promotes innovation and change in medical education. Any plan to publish or disseminate outcomes must consider whether IRB approval or exemption and the protection of learners as human subjects are required. Educators should consider the protection of their intellectual property and become familiar with their university's copyright policy.

What to disseminate may range from curricular content, to a curriculum guide, to outcomes related to the curriculum. What form the scholarly product should take may follow from what is disseminated. In addition to publications, scholarly products may include Web-based materials, textbooks or textbook chapters, teaching modules, continuing medical education presentations, or community education (Fincher et al. 2000). A poster to present at a conference is perhaps the simplest scholarly product (see Singh 2014). Another method is a workshop, symposium, or course at the regional, national, or international conference of a professional medical society; this allows for networking as well as direct feedback (see Spagnoletti et al. 2013). Publication in a peer-reviewed journal is the most time-intensive approach but has the widest reach and longest-lasting impact (see Yager et al. 2018).

Finally, educators should consider submitting scholarly products to one of the Web-based repositories of medical curricula discussed. Because curricula published in MedEdPortal (www.mededportal.org) are peer reviewed, publication should count toward promotion and tenure.

## CONCLUSION

Adopting a scholarly approach to educational projects will help a psychiatric educator develop a more effective curriculum, better anticipate changes and problems, and ultimately contribute to the medical education literature. A scholarly approach includes clearly delineating the problem to be solved, identifying resources to help solve the problem, conducting a needs assessment, determining what the intended outcome should be, selecting the appropriate method of intervention, implementing the intervention, measuring the outcome, and using the outcome to inform future interventions. The educator should be culturally sensitive to ensure that the clinical learning environment is inclusive for learners, teachers, patients, and all other stakeholders. A scholarly approach also serves as a prerequisite for educational scholarship and research, which includes disseminating the outcome of the educational project.

## REFERENCES

Accreditation Council for Graduate Medical Education: Accreditation (website). Accreditation Council for Graduate Medical Education, 2019. Available at: https://www.acgme.org/Program-Directors-and-Coordinators/Welcome/Accreditation. Accessed September 14, 2019.

American Psychiatric Association: Diagnostic and Statistical Manual of Mental Disorders, 5th Edition. Arlington, VA, American Psychiatric Association, 2013

Anderson LW, Krathwohl DR, Airasian PW: A Taxonomy for Learning, Teaching, and Assessing: A Revision of Bloom's Taxonomy of Educational Objectives. New York, Longman, 2001

Association of American Medical Colleges: Research in Medical Education: A Primer for Medical Students. Washington, DC, Association of American Medical Colleges, 2015. Available at: https://www.aamc.org/system/files/c/2/429856-mededresearchprimer.pdf. Accessed September 29, 2019.

Association of American Medical Colleges: CI Physician Competency Reference Set (website). Association of American Medical Colleges, 2019. Available at: https://www.aamc.org/initiatives/cir/establishci/348808/aboutpcrs.html. Accessed September 14, 2019.

Beckman TJ, Cook DA: Developing scholarly projects in education: a primer for medical teachers. Med Teach 29(2–3):210–218, 2007

Best Evidence in Medical Education Collaboration: Published reviews (website). Best Evidence in Medical Education, 2019. Available at: https://www.bemecollaboration.org/Published+Reviews. Accessed October 5, 2019.

Brottman MR, Char DM, Hattori RA, et al: Toward cultural competency in health care: a scoping review of the diversity and inclusion education literature. Acad Med 95(5):803–813, 2020

Dyrbye LN, Thomas MR, Mechaber AJ, et al: Medical education research and IRB review: an analysis and comparison of the IRB review process at six institutions. Acad Med 82(7):654–660, 2007

Englander R, Cameron T, Ballard A, et al: Toward a common taxonomy of competency domains for the health professions and competencies for physicians. Acad Med 88(8):1088–1094, 2013

Fincher RM, Simpson DE, Mennin SP, et al: Scholarship in teaching: an imperative for the 21st century. Acad Med 75(9):887–894, 2000

Gruppen LD, Durning SJ: Needles and haystacks: finding funding for medical education research. Acad Med 91(4):480–484, 2016

Haig A, Dozier M: BEME guide no. 3: systematic searching for evidence in medical education. Part 2: constructing searches. Med Teach 25(5):463–484, 2003

Kaufman DM: Applying educational theory in practice. BMJ 326(7382):213–217, 2003

Liaison Committee on Medical Education: Accreditation prep (website). Liaison Committee on Medical Education, 2019. Available at: http://lcme.org/accreditation-preparation/schools. Accessed September 16, 2019.

Psychiatry Milestone Group: The Psychiatry Milestone Project. Chicago, IL, Accreditation Council for Graduate Medical Education, July 2015. Available at: https://www.acgme.org/Portals/0/PDFs/Milestones/PsychiatryMilestones.pdf?ver=2015-11-06-120520-753. Accessed September 14, 2019.

Reed DA, Cook DA, Beckman TJ, et al: Association between funding and quality of published medical education research. JAMA 298(9):1002–1009, 2007

Roberts LW, Coverdale J, Edenharder K, Louie A: How to review a manuscript: a "down-to-earth" approach. Acad Psychiatry 28(2):81–87, 2004

Sargeant J: Qualitative research, part II: participants, analysis, and quality assurance. J Grad Med Educ 4(1):1–3, 2012

Schwartz A, Young R, Hicks PJ: Medical education practice-based research networks: facilitating collaborative research. Med Teach 38(1):64–74, 2016

Simpson D, Yarris LM, Carek PJ: Defining the scholarly and scholarship common program requirements. J Grad Med Educ 5(4):539–540, 2013

Singh MK: Preparing and presenting effective abstracts and posters in psychiatry. Acad Psychiatry 38(6):709–715, 2014

Spagnoletti CL, Spencer AL, Bonnema RA, et al: Workshop preparation and presentation: a valuable form of scholarship for the clinician-educator. J Grad Med Educ 5(1):155–156, 2013

Sullivan GM: Education research and human subject protection: crossing the IRB quagmire. J Grad Med Educ 3(1):1–4, 2011a
Sullivan GM: Getting off the "gold standard": randomized controlled trials and education research. J Grad Med Educ 3(3):285–289, 2011b
Sullivan GM: Resources for clinicians becoming clinician educators. J Grad Med Educ 7(2):153–155, 2015
Sullivan GM: A toolkit for medical education scholarship. J Grad Med Educ 10(1):1–5, 2018
Sullivan GM, Sargeant J: Qualities of qualitative research: part I. J Grad Med Educ 3(4):449–452, 2011
Thomas P, Kern D, Hughes M, Chen B: Curriculum Development for Medical Education: A Six-Step Approach, 3rd Edition. Baltimore, MD, Johns Hopkins University Press, 2016
Trinh N, Chen J: Sociocultural Issues in Psychiatry: A Casebook and Curriculum. New York, Oxford University Press, 2019
Yager J, Ritvo A, Wolfe JH, Feinstein RE: A survival guide to low-resource peer-reviewed creative scholarship for aspiring clinician-educators. Acad Psychiatry 42(6):841–846, 2018

## CHAPTER 6

# ENHANCING DIVERSITY AND INCLUSION IN PSYCHIATRY TRAINING

Vishal Madaan, M.D.
Adrienne Adams, M.D., M.S.
Colin Stewart, M.D.
Francis Lu, M.D.

**While** society continues to become more inclusive, diversity in medicine—especially academic medicine—lags behind. As a catalyst for health equity, a diverse physician workforce not only is about creating fairness but also has measurable benefits, including higher patient satisfaction and trust. Diversity encompasses much more than ethnicity and race and includes gender, sexual orientation, age, socioeconomic status, and religious/spiritual associations (Ton and Lim 2015).

The need for and impact of diversity in the physician workforce was recognized in 2009 with the creation of the Liaison Committee on Medical Education (LCME) accreditation standard on diversity and inclusion for U.S. and Canadian medical schools:

> **Standard 3: Academic and Learning Environments**
> A medical school ensures that its medical education program occurs in professional, respectful, and intellectually stimulating academic and

clinical environments, recognizes the benefits of diversity, and promotes students' attainment of competencies required of future physicians (Liaison Committee on Medical Education 2019, p. 4).

**3.3 Diversity/Pipeline Programs and Partnerships**
A medical school has effective policies and practices in place, and engages in ongoing, systematic, and focused recruitment and retention activities, to achieve mission-appropriate diversity outcomes among its students, faculty, senior administrative staff, and other relevant members of its academic community. These activities include the use of programs and/or partnerships aimed at achieving diversity among qualified applicants for medical school admission and the evaluation of program and partnership outcomes. (Liaison Committee on Medical Education 2019, p. 4)

The Association of American Medical Colleges (AAMC) created the Group on Diversity and Inclusion (www.aamc.org/members/gdi) in 2009 to help medical schools fulfill the LCME accreditation standard. Each medical school has one or more designated "Group on Diversity and Inclusion Officers" who work with the designated officer(s) of the Group on Women in Medicine and Science. The national priorities of this group include diversity and inclusion in faculty, graduate medical education (GME), and professional development/institutional climates.

The Accreditation Council for Graduate Medical Education (ACGME) revision of the Common Program Requirements (CPR) for residency and fellowship training programs effective July 1, 2019, included a CPR on diversity and inclusion for the first time (Accreditation Council for Graduate Medical Education 2018, 2019a). Organizations such as the American Psychiatric Association, the AAMC, and the American Association of Directors of Psychiatric Residency Training (AADPRT) advocated for this new accreditation standard. The specific diversity and inclusion accreditation standard is as follows (Accreditation Council for Graduate Medical Education 2018):

**I.C.** The program, in partnership with its Sponsoring Institution, must engage in practices that focus on mission-driven, ongoing, systematic recruitment and retention of a diverse and inclusive workforce of residents, fellows (if present), faculty members, senior administrative staff members, and other relevant members of its academic community. (Core)

**Background and Intent:** It is expected that the Sponsoring Institution has, and programs implement, policies and procedures related to recruitment and retention of minorities underrepresented in medicine and medical leadership in accordance with the Sponsoring Institution's mission and aims. The program's annual evaluation must include an assessment of the program's efforts to recruit and retain a diverse workforce, as noted in V.C.1.(c).(5).(c).

This action closed the gap between the ACGME standards for all residency and fellowship training programs of all specialties in the United States and the 2009 LCME accreditation standard on diversity and inclusion for U.S. and Canadian medical schools. Furthermore, the AAMC has put forth these definitions of *diversity* and *inclusion* that show the interrelationship between both concepts (Association of American Medical Colleges 2019a):

> **Diversity** as a core value embodies inclusiveness, mutual respect, and multiple perspectives and serves as a catalyst for change resulting in health equity. In this context, we are mindful of all aspects of human differences such as socioeconomic status, race, ethnicity, language, nationality, sex, gender identity, sexual orientation, religion, geography, disability and age.
>
> **Inclusion** is a core element for successfully achieving diversity. Inclusion is achieved by nurturing the climate and culture of the institution through professional development, education, policy, and practice. The objective is creating a climate that fosters belonging, respect, and value for all and encourages engagement and connection throughout the institution and community.

In this chapter, we review current demographic data related to diversity in residency training, illustrate the impact of international medical graduates (IMGs) on diversity in psychiatry residency training, and offer the utility of the holistic review model to enhance diversity and inclusion in GME recruitment.

## THE CONTEXT

Many national organizations and government agencies recognize the problematic lack of diversity in academia and have undertaken various initiatives to promote diversity and inclusion. Measures have been proposed at institutional levels to make the health profession workforce more representative of the population and to reduce health care disparities (Sullivan 2003). The appointment of a chief diversity officer by the ACGME was a good step in promoting diversity initiatives in residency training.

### Current Data Regarding Diversity in Psychiatry

The AAMC, with additional data from the American Medical Association, tracks demographics regarding students entering psychiatry train-

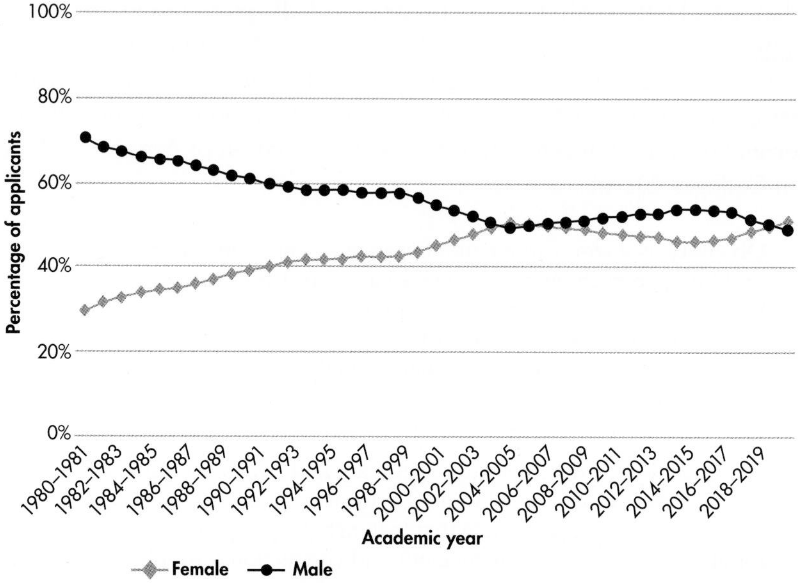


**Figure 6–1. Percentage of applicants to U.S. medical schools by sex, academic years 1980–1981 through 2018–2019.**

Figure excludes applicants who did not report sex.

*Source.* Association of American Medical Colleges (2020b).

ing. Recent data show that females enter psychiatry at approximately the same rate as males, thereby reducing the gender gap and enhancing diversity (Figure 6–1). However, Figure 6–2, which shows ethnicity and race, reflects no growth for Hispanics and African Americans after adjusting for population growth (Association of American Medical Colleges 2019a).

The AADPRT founded a Diversity and Inclusion Committee in 2017, with a mission statement that includes

- Developing and implementing ongoing education in diversity and inclusion for the membership to benefit training programs both general and subspecialties nationally.
- Collaborating with other committees on promoting diversity and inclusion within the leadership of the organization and encouraging recruitment and retention in academic settings.
- Partnering with committees already in existence to advocate for issues about diversity and health care disparities.

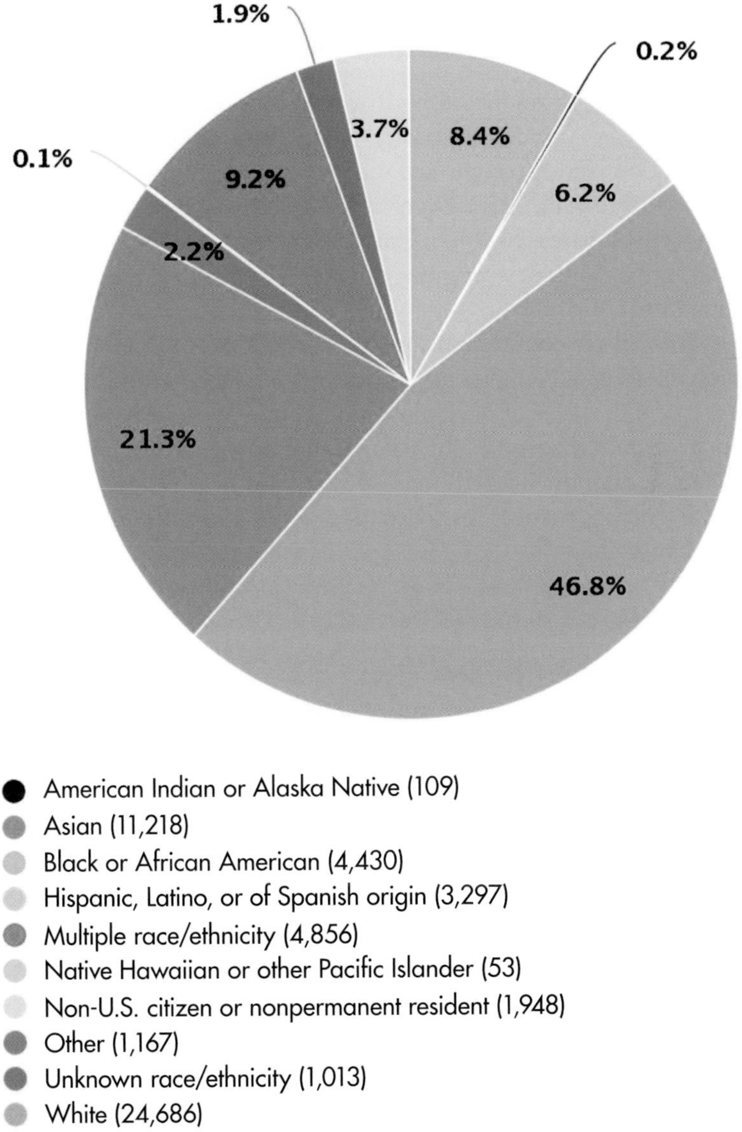


**Figure 6–2. Percentage of applicants to U.S. medical schools by race/ethnicity (alone), academic year 2018–2019. (See Plate 1 to view this figure in color.)**

Race/Ethnicity "alone" indicates that an individual is reported in only one race/ethnicity category. The "Multiple race/ethnicity" category includes individuals who selected more than one race/ethnicity response. The "Non-U.S. citizen or nonpermanent resident" category may include individuals with unknown citizenship.

*Source.* Association of American Medical Colleges (2020a).

With the intent of improving diversity and inclusion in psychiatry educational leadership, the committee examined the AADPRT membership in 2019. Figures 6–3 through 6–7 reflect the findings of that study (Adams 2019).

Previous efforts to increase diversity in undergraduate medical training, such as "population parity" and "Project 3000 by 2000," were aspirational but did not complete the promise of complete diversity in academia (Pierre et al. 2017). Diversity and inclusion remain highly valued in order to address health disparities and health equity (Nivet 2011).

Although a residency program director may believe that diversity is a personal responsibility, diversity and inclusion requirements must be implemented by the entire department. Per ACGME, the sponsoring institution must have "policies and procedures related to recruitment and retention of minorities underrepresented in medicine and medical leadership in accordance with the sponsoring institution's mission and aims" (Accreditation Council for Graduate Medical Education 2019b). Thus, the starting point is an action plan with commitment from institutional leadership.

## Action Plan

The first step is to review the CPR to assess your program's needs for compliance with the diversity and inclusion requirements. The designated institutional officer within the GME department should have current policies on diversity and inclusion in graduate training. Others with this responsibility, such as a chief diversity officer, officers within institutional diversity and inclusion committees, or associate or assistant deans, may also be good sources of information. Such consultations will help you understand the current diversity and inclusion efforts within your institution. Other responsible individuals may provide in-service trainings on selected diversity and inclusion topics or act as a consultant to your department. Your chairperson may develop a diversity advisory committee consisting of faculty and house staff from a broad range of levels. The committee chairperson should be senior level and directly report to the department chair or vice chair (Lu and Adams 2019). The diversity advisory committee should establish core objectives, including

- Establishing infrastructure: meeting frequency, subcommittees, annual retreat, annual report
- Creating a strategic plan for department diversity and inclusion to meet the new CPR
- Establishing guidelines for diverse and inclusive recruitment on residency and fellowship selection committees and faculty search committees

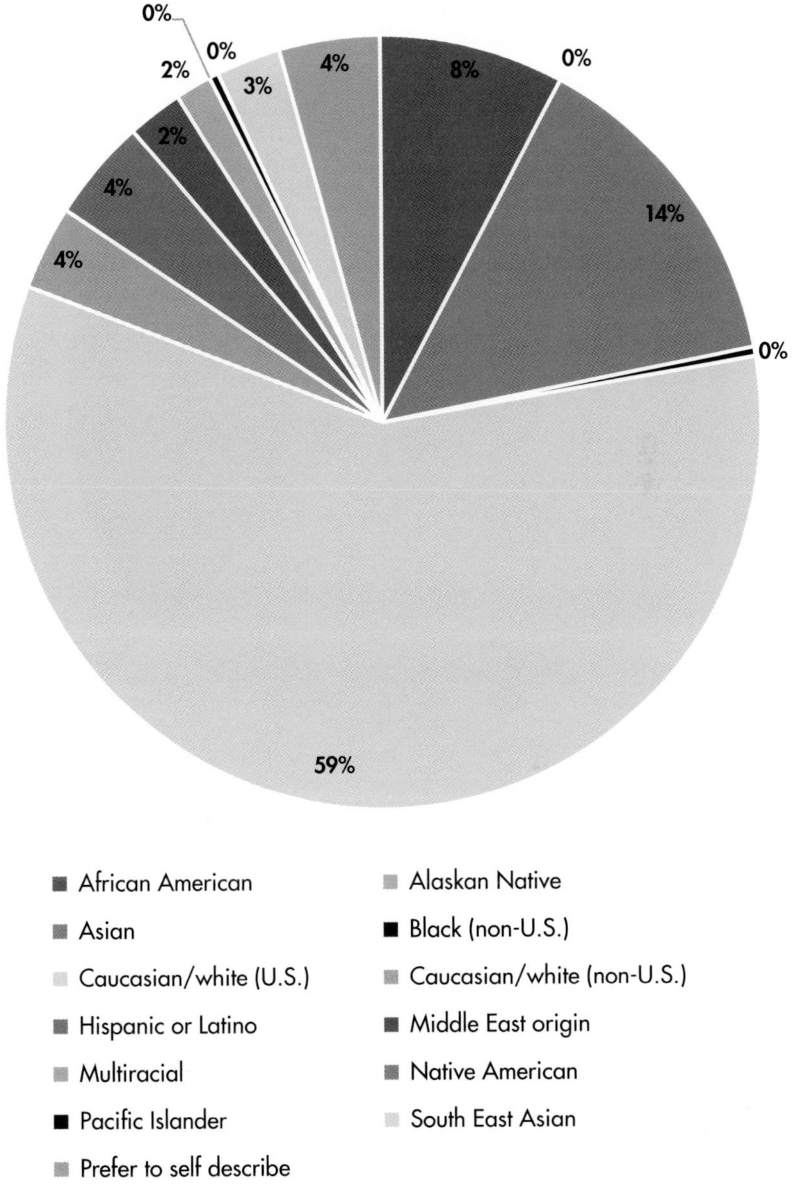


**Figure 6–3. American Association of Directors of Psychiatric Residency Training survey on diversity—membership: Which race/ethnicity best describes you? (See Plate 2 to view this figure in color.)**

*Source.* Adams 2019.

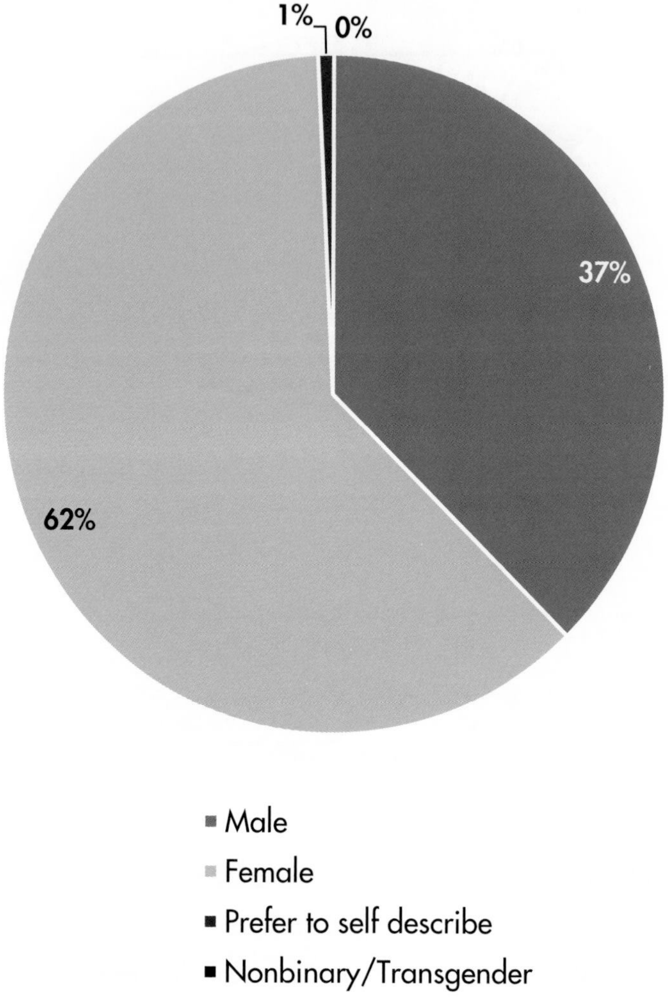


**Figure 6–4. American Association of Directors of Psychiatric Residency Training survey on diversity—membership: What is your gender identity?**
*Source.* Adams 2019.

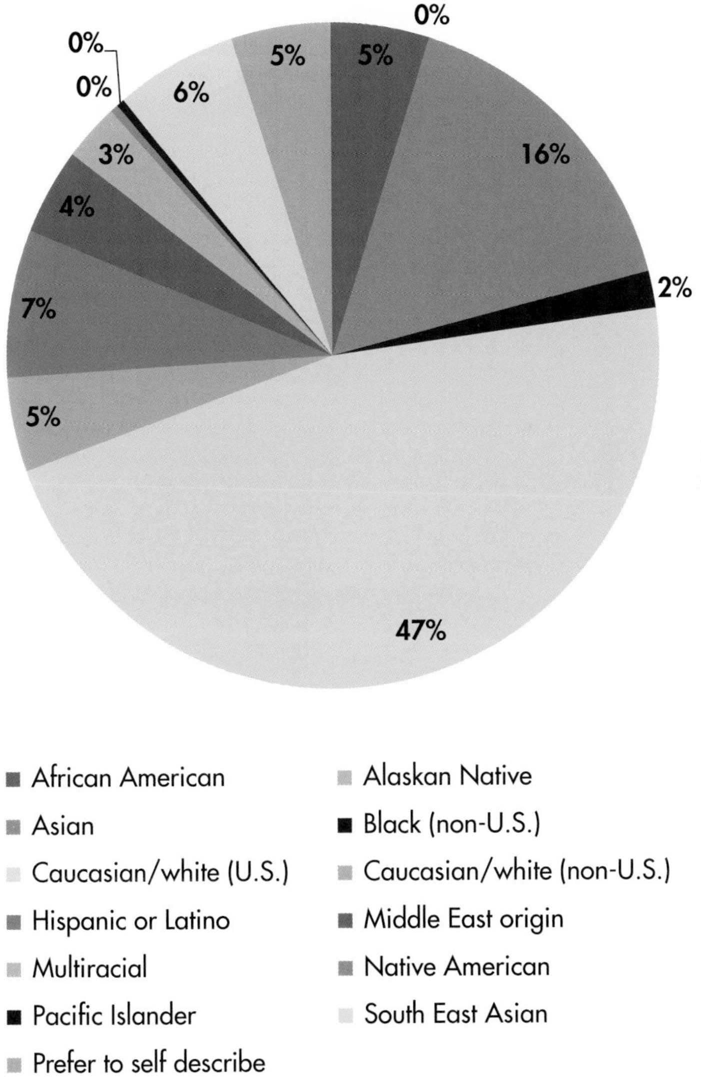


**Figure 6–5. American Association of Directors of Psychiatric Residency Training survey on diversity—trainees: Which race/ethnicity best describes you? (See Plate 3 to view this figure in color.)**

*Source.* Adams 2019.

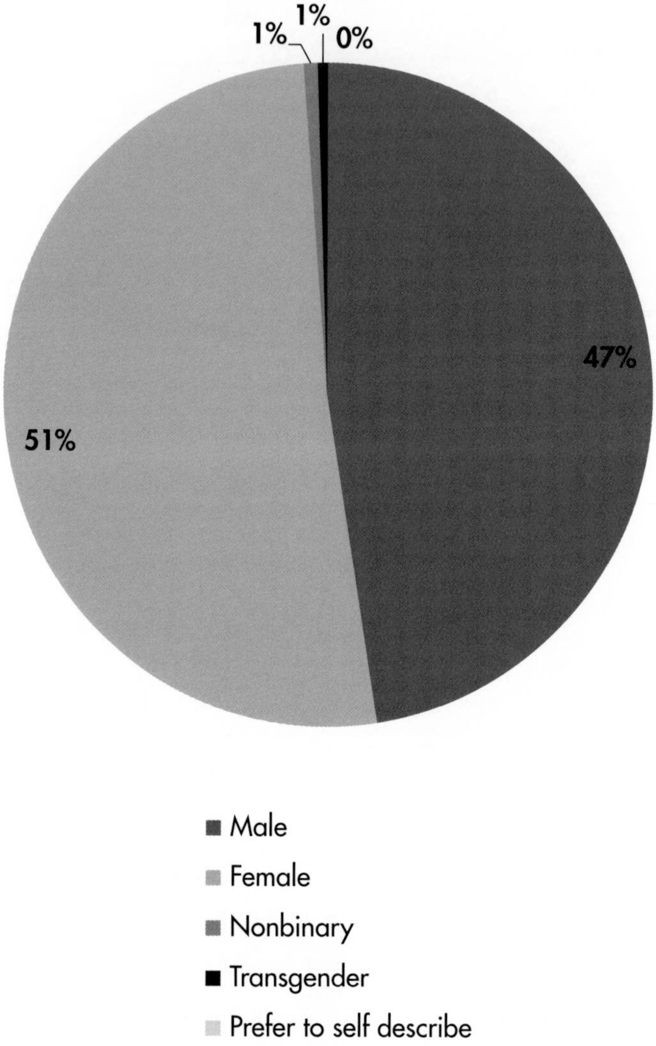


**Figure 6–6. American Association of Directors of Psychiatric Residency Training survey on diversity—trainees: What is your gender identity? (See Plate 4 to view this figure in color.)**

*Source.* Adams 2019.

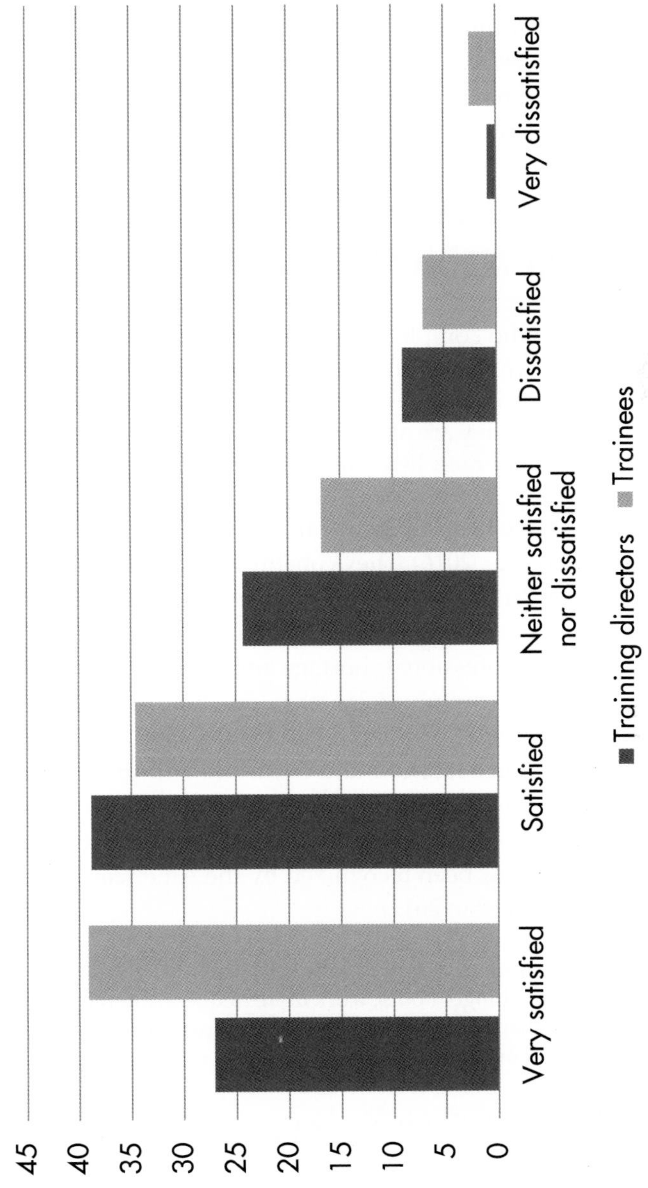


**Figure 6–7.** **Training directors' and trainees' levels of satisfaction with diversity and inclusion efforts in training programs.**
*Source.* Adams 2019.

- Requiring annual evaluation of the program's efforts to recruit and retain a diverse workforce
- Developing diversity initiatives such as
  - Career mentoring programs for early career faculty and trainees
  - Participation in admissions committees
  - Sponsoring discussions on the impact of diversity on health care (i.e., how to minimize unconscious or implicit bias in recruitment)
  - Creating a welcoming and inclusive climate

## THE CURIOUS CASE OF THE INTERNATIONAL MEDICAL GRADUATE

IMGs are physicians who complete medical school outside the United States and pursue or complete their residency training inside the United States. They are categorized as either foreign or U.S. IMGs based on their citizenship status. They are of diverse ethnic, national, and cultural identities, independent of race. IMGs train in more than 2,500 academic programs in more than 150 countries throughout the world.

IMG physicians have been an essential component of the U.S. physician workforce (Rao et al. 2016). They constitute about 30% of the psychiatric workforce, including similar percentages in child and geriatric psychiatry. Studies have demonstrated that IMG physicians are more concentrated in health professional shortage areas and areas with lower per-capita income and a low physician-to-population ratio (Mick and Lee 1996; Polsky et al. 2002). Similarly, IMG physicians treat a higher proportion of patients on Medicaid and Medicare and treat more patients from ethnic and racial minority groups (Ranasinghe 2015).

The significance of work done by IMG psychiatrists in treating underserved populations has been recognized by the American Psychiatric Association (Jeste and Rao 2012):

> IMGs play a critical role in caring for the underserved. Studies have shown that IMGs work longer hours, work more frequently in the public sector, and treat a higher proportion of patients with psychotic disorders than USMGs [U.S. medical graduates]. IMGs also receive a higher percentage of their income from Medicaid and Medicare than do USMGs, the reverse being true for self-payment by patients. Therefore, policies that substantially decrease the availability of IMG psychiatrists may adversely affect the care of minorities and other underserved populations.

With the continued growth in the U.S. minority population, the need for diversity among physicians has never been greater. The LCME, the

ACGME, and institutional stakeholders have recognized this essential need and emphasized measures to enhance diversity in training programs but as yet have overlooked IMGs as a source of such diversity. IMGs bring essential skills, especially in culture-informed syndromes and culture-based approaches to psychopharmacology and individual and family psychotherapy. Although sometimes appreciated as a valuable resource, IMGs may be subjected to unfairness, negative perceptions, mockery, exploitation, and, at times, frank discrimination (Pumariega et al. 2016). Such mixed experiences can serve as obstacles to their personal and professional growth. In addition, separation from family of origin, acculturation, communication issues, working in different health care hierarchies, and visa concerns add to experiences that test their resilience.

The growing number of U.S. medical school graduates with M.D. and D.O. degrees, with no corresponding increase in accredited residency positions, has resulted in fewer IMGs in psychiatry training. U.S. graduates apply to an exponentially higher number of residency programs, which limits interview slots, regardless of their plans to actually interview with or join a particular residency. These recent changes, along with trends suggesting that IMGs may be reconsidering GME in the United States, will not favorably impact the health care of a diverse and growing U.S. population (Boulet et al. 2012). A recent review of National Residency Matching Program postgraduate year-1 psychiatry data suggested a decrease in IMG numbers from about 30% in 2014 to approximately 17% in 2019 (Khan et al. 2019). This downward trend will greatly affect subspecialty training, where IMGs constitute even more sizable numbers.

Successful efforts in diversity and inclusion in GME must include meritocratic recruitment and retention of IMGs. This requires strong commitment from institutional and national education leaders, including program directors, designated institutional officials, and deans of medical schools. IMG applicants must undergo equivalent programmatic scrutiny and not be excluded on the basis of visa paperwork or lack of understanding of cultural norms. More opportunities for observerships should exist to make IMGs more familiar with the U.S. health care system. Interviews with IMG faculty are highly recommended. IMG residents greatly benefit from having a mixture of mentors and supervisors—some with similar backgrounds who can guide them by sharing personal experiences of navigating personal and professional dilemmas, and some from the United States who can train them about the nuances of clinical experiences. Structured feedback and hands-on mentorship, along with program director understanding of personal challenges, visa issues, and acculturation dilemmas, are essential for nurturing IMG residents (Pierre et al. 2017). Successful and sustained integration of IMGs enhances diversity in training programs and, in essence, allows for holistic growth and development within a program.

## HOLISTIC REVIEW: A COMPREHENSIVE APPROACH TO INCREASING DIVERSITY AND INCLUSION AND PROMOTING EQUITY IN THE GME RECRUITMENT PROCESS

### Defining Holistic Review

Holistic review is a key method to promote diversity, inclusion, and equity in recruitment. The AAMC defines *holistic review* in medical education as

> a flexible, highly individualized process by which balanced consideration is given to the multiple ways in which applicants may prepare for and demonstrate suitability as medical students and future physicians. Under a holistic review framework, candidates are evaluated by criteria that are "institution-specific, broad-based, and mission-driven and that are applied equitably across the entire candidate pool." (Association of American Medical Colleges 2010, p. ix)

Selection committees utilizing holistic review begin by defining the core mission, values, and goals of the training program. This process involves considering the needs of the local patient population, the institution, and the field of psychiatry. The selection committee then uses the defined institutional mission, values, and goals as guideposts for selection criteria.

Criteria linked to these guideposts necessarily encompass a broader range of factors than typical review processes. This is intentional, because a broad range of criteria is necessary to capture the unique humanity and life experiences of a more diverse applicant pool. The same selection criteria are used during each step of the recruitment process, and the committee reviews each applicant using these criteria in a structured manner.

### Why Holistic Review?

Holistic review addresses two key elements of the new ACGME core requirement that programs and departments recruit and retain trainees, faculty, and staff members from underrepresented groups. First, it addresses the need for a set of "policies and procedures" oriented toward promoting diversity and inclusion in recruitment because it is a comprehensive set of processes easily codified into policies and outlined as procedures (Accreditation Council for Graduate Medical Education 2018, p. 5). Second, holistic review explicitly orients those policies and procedures around the institution's mission and aims.

Holistic review also offers the advantage of providing a comprehensive framework for recruitment that psychiatry departments can apply not only to trainees but also to "faculty members, senior administrative staff members, and other relevant members of its academic community" included in the new CPR (Accreditation Council for Graduate Medical Education 2018, p. 5). Although structured, this recruitment method is easily modified by different recruitment teams within the department to meet the unique needs of each of these important groups of employees.

In addition to meeting regulatory standards, holistic review may increase a sense of equity and justice in departmental recruitment processes. Burnout among historically excluded and underrepresented groups in medicine might thus be reduced, because there is a correlation between a lower sense of organizational justice and higher rates of burnout (Liljegren and Ekberg 2009). Another benefit of holistic review, applied appropriately, is that it meets legal muster for the use of race or ethnicity as a factor in the selection process. The use of race and ethnicity in the selection process must be "aligned with mission-related educational interests and goals associated with student diversity; and when considered as a broader mix of factors, which may include personal attributes, experiential factors, demographics, or other considerations" (Association of American Medical Colleges 2019b). This is in accordance with federal law and as permitted by state law.

## Support From the Literature

Finally, a growing literature supports holistic review as a means to increase the diversity of both the applicant pool and the trainees matched into undergraduate medical education (UME) and GME (Grabowski 2018; Grbic et al. 2019). Specifically, increases in the racial and ethnic diversity of applicants and matriculants have been documented, as well as increases in the number of students who were the first in their family to attend college in medical schools that adopted holistic review (Grbic et al. 2019). The internal medicine program at the McGovern Medical School at the University of Texas Health Science Center at Houston implemented holistic review in academic year 2016–2017 and immediately saw an increase in the number of applicants, students interviewed, and students who matriculated into GME who were from groups underrepresented in medicine (Aibana et al. 2019).

## Implementing Holistic Review at Your Institution

Programs developing holistic review at their institutions will need to take the following seven steps:

1. Conduct a needs assessment.
2. Draft mission, values, priorities, and goals.
3. Determine specific, measurable outcomes.
4. Develop selection criteria balancing experiences, attributes, and metrics (EAM).
5. Apply criteria equitably throughout recruitment process.
6. Evaluate outcomes based on original goals.
7. Adjust EAM as needed.

## Conducting a Needs Assessment and Drafting a Mission Statement, Values, Priorities, and Goals

Programs must gather data about the needs of their local patient population, the population they serve from a national perspective, and the field. For example, child and adolescent fellowships should consider the rapidly changing demographic makeup of youth nationally and then learn more about the specific demographics of the patient population in their region. Addiction psychiatry fellowships might take into account which local populations have been hit hardest by the opioid epidemic.

Program leadership should then meet to assess and define core program values. Examples of program values include diversity, inclusion, and equity; curiosity and humility; sense of community responsibility; and the premise that people are doing the best they can with what resources they have. The team must then consider goals for the physicians in their department, which might include decreasing health disparities in the local population, advocating for patients to local policymakers, developing research projects oriented toward relieving the suffering of patients that the department serves, and so forth. Finally, the leadership team prioritizes those values and goals.

The team should then draft a mission statement that encapsulates these values, goals, and priorities. One example is the current mission statement of the MedStar Georgetown University Child and Adolescent Psychiatry Training Program:

> We strive to prevent and alleviate youth mental health problems and promote positive youth mental health in the nation's capital by bringing

> state-of-the-art, research-based psychiatric care that is holistic, family centered, community-based, and culturally attuned to the diverse communities of the Washington region in an effort to build health equity. (MedStar Health 2019)

The drafted mission statement is then distributed to all necessary stakeholders for review and comment. Once a mission statement is finalized, it is used as a guide for developing specific, measurable outcomes.

## Determining Specific, Measurable Outcomes

Delineating a set of desired outcomes at the start of holistic review allows programs to evaluate how effective the process is in helping the program meet its goals. Programs may gather baseline data about performance and compare it with data gathered after initiating holistic review. The AAMC has a document to help medical schools evaluate outcomes after implementing holistic review, and the guidance within is easily translated to GME programs (Association of American Medical Colleges 2013). Programs should develop outcomes that both are specific and measurable and are easily tracked over time, such as the number of graduates who work in community psychiatry, the number of graduates who work with the local population, the number of trainees in specific demographic groups, and the number of trainees who were the first person in their family to attend college.

## Defining Experiences, Attributes, and Metrics

Once the mission statement and outcomes have been determined, they guide development of a wide-ranging, balanced set of EAM to serve as selection criteria. *Experiences* generally encompass the journey a trainee has taken to applying for GME training. Examples used by MedStar Georgetown's Child and Adolescent Psychiatry program include having worked with children and adolescents, scholarly experience, personal use of the public health system, growing up in an underserved area, volunteer work with children or the underserved, or extra psychotherapy training.

*Attributes* are considered applicants' "skills and abilities at time of entry to medical school, personal and professional characteristics, and demographic factors" (Association of American Medical Colleges 2010). Examples used by Georgetown's program include leadership skills, Spanish-language skills, ability to maintain professional boundaries, the capacity for self-reflection, intellectual curiosity, empathy, and African American/Black or Latinx ethnicity.

*Metrics* generally include the quantitative components of the application, such as medical school grade point average and examination scores.

**Table 6–1.** Holistic review

| Applicant experience or attribute | Applicant data element(s) |
|---|---|
| Evidence of life experience that would help fulfill our program mission | Personal statement, recommendation letters, curriculum vitae, interviews |
| Community psychiatry experience | Curriculum vitae, residency block schedule |
| Sophisticated empathic capacity | Personal statement, responses to behavioral interview questions |
| Established process for self-reflection | Personal statement, recommendation letters, responses to behavioral interview questions |
| Leadership experience | Curriculum vitae, recommendation letters |

These EAM then are mapped onto available application materials. See Table 6–1 for an example of how MedStar Georgetown University's program translated EAM into available applicant data elements.

## Applying Experiences, Attributes, and Metrics Criteria Equitably Throughout Recruitment

### *SCREENING*

The initial phase of recruitment involves screening submitted applications and choosing applicants to interview. This is generally one of the most time-consuming, frustrating, and challenging tasks for programs because the number of applications received is typically quite large compared with the number of spots to be filled. Program directors struggle to logically and fairly narrow the applicant pool. Most programs settle on a "metrics-first" approach that prioritizes U.S. Medical Licensing Examination (USMLE) Step scores as a cutoff. Fortunately, holistic review can bring both more structure and more equity to this otherwise very difficult process.

The internal medicine residency program at the McGovern Medical School in Houston offers a model for how to manage a large number of applications (approximately 3,500 annually) (Aibana et al. 2019). The program chose to continue a metrics-first approach to determine the initial pool of applicants to interview and then evaluated all applicants who scored ≤10 points below the USMLE cutoff score using predetermined, mission-aligned EAM. Each applicant reviewed in this way received an experience/attribute score; those who scored above a predetermined cutoff were invited to interview. With this methodology, the program increased the proportion of underrepresented minority applicants interviewed by 8.5% and residents matriculating by 19.2% (Aibana et al. 2019).

Fellowship programs may be able to use an experience/attribute-first approach, given that they typically receive many fewer applications than general psychiatry residencies. For example, in the MedStar Georgetown University child and adolescent psychiatry fellowship program, selection committee application reviewers are blinded to applicant metrics when determining who to invite to interview, and applicants are initially ranked based on their experience/attribute score. Online surveys can be a helpful method for collecting and comparing EAM scores.

All faculty reviewing applications should receive training on how to convert application materials into the program's chosen scoring system to improve interrater reliability. Faculty benefit from training about the impact of implicit bias in letter of recommendation letter writing and curriculum vitae development, which should be considered when developing the predetermined experience/attribute scoring system and when reviewing individual applications.

#### *INTERVIEWING*

Interviewing is another area significantly influenced by implicit bias and lack of interrater reliability. Interviews are often the phase of recruitment in which faculty feel most comfortable and confident; at the same time, it is generally the least consistent and least equitable step in applicant review. Fortunately, methods to decrease inconsistency and implicit bias are available. A significant literature supports using structured or semistructured interviews conducted by two or more faculty members to increase the reliability and validity of interviewers' judgments (Harasym et al. 1996).

Behavioral interviewing focuses on thoughtfully designing questions that assess specific experiences and attributes. The Vanderbilt University anesthesiology residency program aligned behavioral interview questions with ACGME core competencies (Easdown et al. 2005). The MedStar Georgetown University fellowship adjusted this model to incorporate questions that assess both holistic review–derived attributes and competencies from the ACGME milestones. For example, one question assessed the attribute of "sophisticated empathic capacity" and the overlapping competency area of "compassion, integrity, respect for others, sensitivity to diverse patient populations, adherence to ethical principles" by asking, "How have you connected with patients who are different from yourself?" As in the screening phase, online surveys may be helpful in compiling experience/attribute scores based on data collected during individual interviews.

### *RANKING*

In the final step of the recruitment process, data collected from the previous steps are gathered and evaluated by the selection committee. The selection committee is ideally composed using a holistic review process of the kind being piloted at Baylor University School of Medicine for both recruitment and advancement of faculty (Harris et al. 2018). Such a process may ensure sufficient diversity of perspectives to identify and account for potential biases during screening, interviewing, and ranking. Committees should determine point values for each EAM prior to the start of recruitment for final ranking.

## Evaluating Outcomes

After the recruitment and selection processes are complete, programs should shift their focus to collecting and sorting outcome data. Collecting data might include surveying faculty about their experience during the holistic review process, surveying applicants about their experience during recruitment, and evaluating applicant-related data available after the end of interviews (e.g., applicant ethnicity). Surveys may be conducted at the end of the academic year to assess outcomes related to the program learning environment, and surveys targeted toward graduates might assess outcomes related to postgraduation work placement.

## Transparency and Authenticity

The transition to holistic review may incur resistance from trainees, faculty, and staff. Program directors must communicate the process and goals clearly. Effective messaging should consistently tie these changes to the program mission, values, and goals and illustrate the advantages of increasing diversity. Communication about the holistic review process on program website materials and in the interview-day orientation may play a valuable role in helping develop a greater sense of inclusion for applicants.

## Final Considerations: Holistic Review 2.0

Because GME is early in the process of using holistic review, much still needs to be done regarding research and tailoring the processes and procedures developed in UME for GME. One important area is analyzing the performance of past trainees to determine which EAM are most predictive of trainee future success both clinically and as related to the mission-related goals mentioned (e.g., serving the local underserved population after graduation or choosing electives aligned with the program's mission). Another area for future research and development would be developing better Likert scales to gather data about screener and interviewer evaluation of applications and applicants that include anchored, more objective descriptions (much like developmental "milestones" descriptions have replaced the Likert-scale designations in the ACGME milestones document).

# CONCLUSION

With growing diversity in the U.S. population, the need for diversity and inclusion in academic medicine has never been greater. Concerted efforts by the LCME to enhance diversity have been ongoing, and the ACGME has more recently begun to further that effort. This requires sustained commitment from institutional and departmental leadership as well as innovative ways to address the lack of diversity. Holistic reviews should be considered to enhance diversity and inclusion and to allow for meaningful and meritocratic ways of recruitment. Similarly, IMG recruitment not only adds to programmatic diversity but also brings in maturity, resilience, and opportunities for enhancing cultural competence.

## — KEY POINTS —

- Patterns of diversity in academia lag behind similar trends in society.
- The Accreditation Council for Graduate Medical Education requirements include one on diversity and inclusion.
- Implementation of diversity and inclusion requirements requires unwavering commitment from the institutional leadership, departmental chairs, and program leadership.
- Successful recruitment of international medical graduates can be an effective and unique way of enhancing diversity in residency training.
- Holistic review is a flexible, individualized, and comprehensive approach to increasing diversity and inclusion and promoting equity in the graduate medical education recruitment process.

# REFERENCES


Accreditation Council for Graduate Medical Education: ACGME Common Program Requirements (Residency). Chicago, IL, Accreditation Council on Graduate Medical Education, 2018. Available at: https://www.acgme.org/Portals/0/PFAssets/ProgramRequirements/CPRResidency2020.pdf and https://www.acgme.org/Portals/0/PFAssets/ProgramRequirements/CPRFellowship2020.pdf. Accessed March 29, 2020.

Accreditation Council for Graduate Medical Education: ACGME names first chief diversity and inclusion officer. ACGME News, March 11, 2019a. Available at: https://www.acgme.org/Newsroom/Newsroom-Details/articleId/8038. Accessed October 30, 2019.

Accreditation Council for Graduate Medical Education: Common Program Requirements (website). Accreditation Council on Graduate Medical Education, 2019b. Available at: https://www.acgme.org/What-We-Do/Accreditation/Common-Program-Requirements. Accessed October 30, 2019.

Adams A: AADPRT's perspective on diversity and inclusion in CLER: the role of national organizations. Presented at the annual meeting of the American Psychiatric Association, San Francisco, CA, 2019

Aibana O, Swails JL, Flores RJ, Love L: Bridging the gap: holistic review to increase diversity in graduate medical education. Acad Med 94(8):1137–1141, 2019

Association of American Medical Colleges: Roadmap to Diversity: Integrating Holistic Review Practices Into Medical School Admission Processes. Washington, DC, Association of American Medical Colleges, 2010

Association of American Medical Colleges: Roadmap to Excellence: Key Concepts for Evaluating the Impact of Medical School Holistic Admissions. Washington, DC, Association of American Medical Colleges, 2013

Association of American Medical Colleges: Group on Diversity and Inclusion (website). Association of American Medical Colleges, 2019a. Available at: https://www.aamc.org/professional-development/affinity-groups/gdi. Accessed October 30, 2019.

Association of American Medical Colleges: Holistic review. AAMC website, 2019b. Available at: https://www.aamc.org/services/member-capacity-building/holistic-review. Accessed November 1, 2019.

Association of American Medical Colleges: Percentage of applicants to U.S. medical schools by race/ethnicity (alone), academic year 2018-2019. Diversity in Medicine: Facts and Figures. AAMC website, 2020a. Available at: https://www.aamc.org/data-reports/workforce/interactive-data/figure-2-percentage-applicants--us-medical-schools-race/ethnicity-alone-academic-year-2018-2019. Accessed January 23, 2020.

Association of American Medical Colleges: Percentage of applicants to U.S. medical schools by sex, academic years 1980-1981 through 2018-2019. Diversity in Medicine: Facts and Figures. AAMC website, 2020b. Available at: https://www.aamc.org/data-reports/workforce/interactive-data/figure-i-percentage-applicants-us medical-schools-sex-academic-years-1980-1981-through-2018-2019. Accessed January 23, 2020.

Boulet JR, Cassimatis EG, Opalek A: The role of international medical graduate psychiatrists in the United States healthcare system. Acad Psychiatry 36:293–299, 2012

Easdown LJ, Castro PL, Shinkle EP, et al: The behavioral interview: a method to evaluate ACGME competencies in resident selection: a pilot project. J Educ Perioper Med 7(1):E032, 2005

Grabowski CJ: Impact of holistic review on student interview pool diversity. Adv Health Sci Educ Theory Practice 23(3):487–498, 2018

Grbic D, Morrison E, Sondheimer HM, et al: The association between a holistic review in admissions workshop and the diversity of accepted applicants and students matriculating to medical school. Acad Med 94(3):396–403, 2019

Harasym PH, Woloschuk W, Mandin H, Brundin-Mather R: Reliability and validity of interviewers' judgments of medical school candidates. Acad Med 71(1 suppl):S40–S42, 1996

Harris TB, Thomson WA, Moreno NP, et al: Advancing holistic review for faculty recruitment and advancement. Acad Med 93(11):1658–1662, 2018

Jeste D, Rao NR: International medical graduates and APA. Psychiatric News, October 5, 2012. Available at: https://psychnews.psychiatryonline.org/doi/full/10.1176/pn.47.19.psychnews_47_19_8-a. Accessed December 17, 2019.

Khan A, Grullon A, Cotes R: Understanding trends and geographic variation among International Medical Graduates using 2014–2018 National Resident Matching Program data. Presented at the AADPRT annual meeting, San Diego, CA, 2019

Liaison Committee on Medical Education: Functions and Structure of a Medical School: Standards for Accreditation of Medical Education Programs Leading to the MD Degree. Washington, DC, Association of American Medical Colleges, 2019. Available at: https://lcme.org/wp-content/uploads/filebase/standards/2020-21_Functions-and-Structure_2019-10-04.docx. Accessed October 30, 2019.

Liljegren M, Ekberg K: The associations between perceived distributive, procedural, and interactional organizational justice, self-rated health and burnout. Work 33(1):43–51, 2009

Lu F, Adams A: ACGME Common Program Requirement (CPR) on diversity and inclusion: how can training programs prepare for July 2019? Presented at the AADPRT annual meeting, San Diego, CA, 2019

MedStar Health: Child and Adolescent Psychiatry Training Program. MedStar website, 2019. Available at: https://www.medstarhealth.org/education/affiliated-hospitals-2/medstar-georgetown-university-hospital/child-and-adolescent-psychiatry-residency. Accessed November 1, 2019.

Mick SS, Lee SYD: An Analysis of the Comparative Distribution of Active Post Resident IMGs and USMGs in the United States in 1996. Report to the Bureau of Health Professions. Rockville, MD, Health Resources and Services Administration, 1996

Nivet M: Commentary: Diversity 3.0: a necessary systems upgrade. Acad Med 86(12):1487–1489, 2011

Pierre J, Mahr F, Carter A, Madaan V: Underrepresented in medicine recruitment: rationale, challenges, and strategies for increasing diversity in psychiatry residency programs. Acad Psychiatry 41(2):226–232, 2017

Polsky D, Kletke PR, Wozniak GD, Escarce JJ: Initial practice locations of international medical graduates. Health Serv Res 37:907–928, 2002

Pumariega A, Cagande C, Gogineni RR: Child and adolescent psychiatry, in International Medical Graduate Physicians: A Guide to Training. Edited by Rao NR, Roberts LW. New York, Springer International, 2016, pp 185–202

Ranasinghe P: International Medical Graduates in the US Physician Workforce. The Journal of the American Osteopathic Association 115:236–241, 2015

Rao NR, Kramer M, Mehra A: The history of international medical graduate physicians in psychiatry and medicine in the United States: a perspective, in International Medical Graduate Physicians: A Guide to Training. Edited by Rao NR, Roberts LW. New York, Springer International, 2016, pp 245–256

Sullivan LJ: Missing Persons: Minorities in the Health Professions. Atlanta, GA, W.K. Kellogg Foundation, 2003

Ton H, Lim RF: Assessment of culturally diverse individuals, in Clinical Manual of Cultural Psychiatry. Edited by Lim R. Washington, DC, American Psychiatric Publishing, 2015, pp 1–37

# PART II

# MEDICAL STUDENT EDUCATION

CHAPTER 7

# UNDERGRADUATE PRECLINICAL CURRICULUM AND PSYCHIATRY CLERKSHIPS

Daniel E. Gih, M.D.
Sheritta Strong, M.D.
Sharon Hammer, M.D.

## UNDERGRADUATE PRECLINICAL CURRICULUM

### Administration of the Preclinical Curriculum

*DUTIES OF THE COURSE DIRECTOR*

Directing a preclinical course in psychiatry is similar to conducting an orchestra. All the instructors blend together to create a symphony composed of key basic-science principles, common psychiatric conditions, psychopharmacology, interview skills, and other important behavioral science topics. As the conductor, the course director ascertains the most important content to teach and subsequently coordinates lectures, small groups, modules, standardized patient interviews, and reading assignments. Therefore, an experienced faculty member should coordinate the

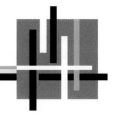

course and integrate the materials taught, prepare and provide lectures, and evaluate other faculty. Nonlecture educational formats may require greater expertise. The course director should meet with any new instructors to orient them and review materials used in teaching.

### *EDUCATIONAL GOALS*

Although many students will not pursue psychiatry as a specialty, they deserve to receive the best psychiatric education possible to prepare them for their clerkships and standardized board examinations and to manage the ubiquity of mental illness in their patients. Because students often view psychiatry as being less scientific than other medical fields, the course leader must provide a neurobiological framework that includes data about the neurobiological effects of psychotherapy in order to create curiosity, further understanding, and enhance validity. The position held by Aparna Iyer, M.D., of modern psychiatry as "part art, all science" (Iyer 2017) is a better paradigm for course leaders than an attitude of "part art, part science."

A well-delivered preclinical curriculum may lead students to further seek out psychiatry faculty or to connect with psychiatry interest groups and national organizations. Early, high-quality exposure decreases the stigma and increases interest in psychiatry (Harper and Roman 2017). Office hours (virtual and live) with the course director may facilitate contact with students for both curriculum-related questions and career exploration.

### *CURRICULUM PLANNING*

The noted education reformer Abraham Flexner understood that medical education reform should evolve with changes in social, political, economic, and scientific areas for subsequent generations in medicine to progress. Fittingly, Flexner's "2+2 medical school model," with preclinical basic science courses and pathophysiology in the first and second year followed by clinical clerkships, is being dismantled as many schools undergo major curriculum reform. Some schools are shortening the preclinical years with better integration of the basic sciences with clinical sciences. Other changes in curricula include a transition from outcome-based education to competency-based courses. This advances self-directed learning and the enhancement of problem-solving skills, a requirement for accreditation by the Liaison Committee on Medical Education (LCME).

Major curricular change requires substantial investment of time and multiple stakeholders' input to make the curriculum more innovative and responsive to current trends. An effective psychiatric curriculum incorporates guidance from consensus materials and guidelines, such as those provided by the National Board of Medical Examiners (NBME), the U.S. Medical Licensing Examination (USMLE), Accreditation Council for Graduate Medical Education (ACGME), American Psychiatric Association, and Association of Directors of Medical Student Education in Psychiatry (ADMSEP).

## Preclinical Course Content and Delivery

### *BEHAVIORAL SCIENCE IN THE PRECLINICAL CURRICULUM*

Little consensus exists on the elements of preclinical behavioral science. Most agree that communication with patients is an essential component of a preclinical behavioral-science curriculum. A systematic review of the ACGME core competencies and LCME standards found that the most commonly taught skill was communication (Carney et al. 2016). The Institute of Medicine (2004) recommended that a behavioral and social science curriculum include 1) mind-body interactions in health and disease, 2) patient behavior, 3) physician role and behavior, 4) physician–patient interactions, 5) social and cultural issues in health care, and 6) health policy and economics.

Preclinical learning goals should incorporate ADMSEP milestones, developed by a task force and based on the ACGME core competencies (Roman et al. 2016). This task force developed these topics with the intent that individual schools further adapt them to their needs. For example, several learning goals are best implemented in the core curriculum and have typically been termed "the doctor–patient relationship." These concepts and skills are generally taught in integrated courses that are usually multidisciplinary and conducted by the medicine department, with active involvement from psychiatry, and provide early exposure to topics such as empathy and medical ethics.

### *TRENDS IN BEHAVIORAL SCIENCES AND CURRICULUM DEVELOPMENT*

A behavioral science course significantly improves performance on that section of the national board examination (Markham 1979), but the number of hours that are devoted to psychiatry and behavioral health in medical school is variable. In 2013, the LCME reiterated the broader concepts of basic science to include behavioral, sociological, and economic subjects while maintaining integration of biomedical science into contemporaneous delivery of knowledge (Brauer and Ferguson 2015). As such, schools are addressing the demand for graduating medical students to possess skills and knowledge in health care policy, population health, and high-value care by including the science of health care delivery in the longitudinal curriculum (Starr et al. 2017).

Since the 1980s, curricular development has included more team-based learning approaches, such as problem-based learning and interprofessional education, or further reorganized topics into systems-based learning with the integration of clinical and basic sciences. Such changes aim to encourage students to begin thinking like doctors from the start of medical school (Harden 1986). Barriers between basic and clinical sciences should shrink. The second Carnegie report (Carnegie II) included a request to improve this integration (Cooke et al. 2010), such that basic science content pertaining to psychiatry and neurosciences courses be jointly determined and that neuroanatomy, neurophysiology, behavioral neurobiology, and some clinical neurology be included in neurosciences courses.

### *DIAGNOSES AS A FRAMEWORK FOR CONTENT*

Developing a course that teaches psychiatric disorders is easier than developing a course in behavioral sciences. DSM should be introduced to students as a tool that psychiatrists and researchers have developed to standardize diagnoses. The challenge is determining which diagnoses listed in the current iteration of DSM should be taught, since all of the defined mental illnesses cannot practically be addressed in the course. The ADMSEP specifies recommended or "key" diagnoses that all medical students should know (Roman et al. 2016). Teaching a limited number of major conditions allows 1) extrapolation that those conditions are among others grouped according to symptom clusters, 2) selective focus on conditions that are seen more commonly and likely to be tested on the NBME and USMLE examinations, and 3) better utilization of clinical expertise in the department.

Additional goals of psychiatric undergraduate medical education are to teach the pathophysiology, biology, and etiology of major mental health conditions and their treatments. As such, the neuroscience department may be an invaluable resource in basic science teaching. Experts in various subspecialties of psychiatry are also good resources if they can translate their knowledge to an appropriate level for preclinical students.

### *TEACHING FORMATS FOR LEARNING*

Integrating basic sciences with clinical content in large classroom activities and small-group learning activities increases students' motivation to learn, process, and focus on essential information (Klement et al. 2016). The most potent learning experience is when students talk to patients with conditions of interest, but logistics often dictate that this happen during clerkships. Video demonstrations illustrating key principles may be used in asynchronous learning formats. Free, peer-reviewed, and open online resources such as the ADMSEP Clinical Simulation Initiative may supplement teaching materials with self-guided interactive modules (Hawa et al. 2017).

Passive information transfer is no longer recommended. Suggested alternatives for large groups include interactive sessions that require advanced preparation from students, frequent questions directed at students, group discussion and case work, and in-class polling to assess formative learning in real time (Schwartzstein and Roberts 2017). See Chapter 1 for an expanded discussion of adult learning principles.

# PSYCHIATRIC CLERKSHIPS

## Administration

### *WHO IS THE CLERKSHIP DIRECTOR?*

The clerkship director is an important leader in the education of medical students on clinical rotations. This individual should have a passion for clinical medical education and student development. The director is the "face" of psychiatry to medical students and may enhance psychiatry's reputation and status. Clerkship directors may be faculty in any stage of their career, but a wealth of clinical practice experience will make for a stronger director. Such experience increases confidence, informs clinical and formal teaching, and enhances student interactions. The director should be an excellent teacher, committed to assuring a high-quality learning experience, and capable of developing faculty teaching skills. Often, the director is a mentor and role model for junior faculty.

These responsibilities may be daunting to a new clerkship director. Mentorship with an outgoing psychiatry clerkship director or a clerkship director from a different academic department may help with the transition into the role. Regular engagement with other directors on a national level is strongly encouraged to learn best practices. ADMSEP is the national organization for psychiatric clerkship directors and other medical student educators and provides support in the form of educational programming, annual meetings, and a national listserv.

Protected time to administer the clerkship is an important consideration for the director and a point of negotiation with the department chair. The amount of protected time given varies by program but generally ranges from 0.4 to 0.5 full-time equivalent value depending on the amount of direct teaching, class size, administrative requirements, and required interactive teaching activities, such as an Objective Structured Clinical Examination. A higher full-time equivalent value has been recognized as appropriate given the teaching and scholarly activities expected by a clerkship director (Pangaro et al. 2003).

### *RESPONSIBILITIES OF THE CLERKSHIP DIRECTOR*

The director must ensure an impactful clinical experience for medical students and fulfill both the LCME requirements for implementing a clinical educational program and the institution's priorities. Additional responsibilities include clerkship site selection; site director orientation and supervision; student site assignments; assessment of site quality and safety; development, implementation, and assessment of didactics; evaluation, examination, and grading of students; remediation of students; career guidance; and feedback. The clerkship director should fully orient new faculty and preceptors in person to the structure, objectives, and grading process for the clerkship.

### *MANAGING CLINICAL SITES AND PRECEPTORS*

Robust clinical services led by engaged site directors with a commitment to education are vital to successful clerkships. Generally, inpatient and consultation-liaison services are the backbone of most psychiatry clerkships. Frequently, the home department will have insufficient academic training sites and personnel; therefore, training sites and additional options for students must be cultivated within the community. There is always a potential risk that training sites or preceptors will be lost due to turnover, program closure, or competing clinical and educational demands. The clerkship director must attend to any personnel changes among community sites.

Site directors are points of contact for the clerkship and responsible for the real-time student learning experience, the teaching environment including preceptors, and the provision of formative and summative feedback to students. An ever-present task for the clerkship director is to identify, recruit, and support site directors. Site directors may be lost to job transitions or retirement.

Nonsalaried community-based psychiatrists who volunteer to teach are primarily motivated by personal satisfaction rather than financial incentives (Kumar et al. 2002). Faculty development, grand rounds or other continuing medical education, complimentary access to online library resources, parking, university-affiliated discounts, or connection with the academic faculty are potential sources of compensation for volunteer faculty (McGeehan et al. 2013). Psychiatrists who are alumni of the clerkship's academic institution are often ideal candidates. A process should be in place to coordinate between the college of medicine and the department of psychiatry to efficiently obtain volunteer faculty status and execute affiliation agreements. The clerkship director should meet periodically with potential or existing volunteer faculty at the clerkship site to get a good overview of the facility and teaching.

### *THE CLERKSHIP COORDINATOR*

Use of educational software by institutions has increased significantly. Thus, clerkship coordinators must be adept with technology. An effective coordinator is a tremendous asset. The coordinator's responsibilities include scheduling and communicating with students about the clerkship, organizing orientation, preparing educational materials, scheduling lectures and reserving classrooms, distributing and collecting evaluations, proctoring examinations, and preparing grades. Coordinators are the first point of contact for students regarding problems or concerns. They communicate regularly with site directors, distribute student feedback, and gather grading information.

Coordinators must be flexible problem solvers because of the many time-sensitive issues that arise, such as student requests for time off, unanticipated absences of site directors, and changes in didactic schedules. Coordinators are often the "heart" of the clerkship, trusted confidantes with whom students can share worries, struggles, and successes during the rotation. It is essential that coordinators be confident and emotionally mature individuals who have a passion for student development.

Regular weekly meetings between the clerkship director and coordinator are recommended. Even when the clerkship appears to be on "autopilot" and running smoothly, these weekly meetings can generate ideas for improving the clerkship and enhancing student learning and can promote a trusting, collegial relationship between the director and coordinator that is essential to a healthy clerkship.

## The Clerkship Experience

### *CLERKSHIP LENGTH*

There has been a trend toward decreasing psychiatry clerkship length. Six weeks is the most common length (49.5%); only 18.9% of clerkships last 8 weeks (Rosenthal et al. 2005). Another trend is combining psychiatry with other clerkships, usually neurology and less frequently internal or family medicine (Clegg 2003). The clerkship director and other key education faculty negotiate the length of the psychiatry clerkship with the college of medicine.

The most cogent argument for retaining or expanding the psychiatry clerkship length is the pressing need for primary care physicians to be well trained in psychiatric diagnosis and treatment. Patients with mental illnesses often receive treatment in primary care; the suffering and cost of inadequate psychiatric diagnosis and treatment are high. The psychiatry clerkship is where most psychiatry training will occur for future primary care physicians because opportunities for psychiatry training in primary care residency vary widely by specialty and program.

An argument cannot be made that shortened psychiatry clerkships adversely affect national standardized assessment measures. Several studies have shown that a reduction in psychiatry clerkship length of up to 50% does not adversely affect the NBME psychiatry subject examination scores or USMLE Step 2 clinical knowledge scores in the mental disorders subsection (Niedermier et al. 2010). What is of concern regarding shortened psychiatry clerkships is that such clerkships rely heavily on the NBME subject examination as their evaluation tool. The result is teaching toward knowledge rather than toward clinical skills because less time is available for direct observation of student interactions with patients or for assessment using standardized evaluations of clinical competency (Rosenthal et al. 2005).

### *ASSIGNMENT OF STUDENTS WITHIN THE ROTATION*

Students may be assigned to single or multiple sites during their clerkship. Students learn most effectively by spending a minimum of 2 weeks at a single site and frequently express a desire to spend a minimum of 3 weeks. Sufficient duration of experience at a site gives students an opportunity to learn how the site functions and to develop rapport with the treatment team and the comfort level to function more independently. Diversity of learning experiences offers students the greatest breadth of knowledge. For instance, a community inpatient site may be paired with an academic hospital consultation-liaison site, or an emergency psychiatry rotation may be paired with an outpatient clinic site. Pairing community sites with academic sites whenever possible provides the widest range of student experience.

The location of student assignment does not appear to affect the acquisition of psychiatric knowledge (as measured by standardized examination score) or to influence students' perceptions of psychiatry as a specialty choice (Bobo et al. 2009). Participation in subspecialty clinics, although enriching and often sought after, does not increase scores on the NBME psychiatry subject examination or clinical performance grades (Retamero and Ramchandani 2013). This information should be reassuring to clerkship directors who have a limited number of sites.

Students often express a desire to "choose" their rotation site assignments, but this is time consuming and challenging. Although students may cite future career interest as a reason for preferring a site, a "hidden agenda" may be more favorable hours, less travel time, or obtaining a site director who has a reputation of being more lenient in grading. Therefore, random site assignment is preferable.

### *ATTAINING EQUIVALENCY BETWEEN CLINICAL SITES*

The LCME 8.7 requirement states "that the medical curriculum includes comparable educational experiences and equivalent methods of assessment across all locations within a given course and clerkship to ensure that all medical students achieve the same medical education program objectives" (Liaison Committee on Medical Education 2019). Thus, sites must have the same learning objectives and experiences designed to achieve the same learning outcomes—that is, they must be comparable, although not identical. The requirement infers that instruction is effective at all sites, that the same criteria are used for evaluation, and that sites are monitored and adjusted as needed to maintain equivalency. Clerkship directors must evaluate sites through regular student and site director feedback and in-person visits. Metrics to consider are the variety and breadth of psychiatric diagnoses, number of patients treated, and student hours spent in active patient care. The clerkship director may further ensure equivalency between sites by conducting the same student orientation, distributing the same manual, and providing the same formal didactic curriculum and assessment strategies for all sites. Monitoring examination scores and grades to ensure even distribution across all training sites provides useful feedback about equivalency.

LCME objective 6.2 also assures equivalency and states that each clerkship should specify the types of patients and clinical conditions that all students must see in order to achieve the objectives of the clinical learning environment. Thus, the clerkship director must specify the disease states or conditions that all students are expected to encounter, and students must document the extent to which they interacted with patients during clinical assessments. Results must be regularly reviewed by the director to ensure that students at all training sites meet this standard. The clerkship director can also use ADMSEP's list of "key diagnoses" as a guide for developing a "patient log" for their clerkship, keeping the unique circumstances and patient populations of their clerkship sites in mind.

### *SELECTIVES AND OTHER ACTIVITIES*

Site directors may consider incorporating "selectives" to the clerkship. These are half- to full-day experiences in specific specialty psychiatry areas chosen by the student. Examples include participation in electroconvulsive therapy or other interventional psychiatry treatment, addictions treatment, geriatric psychiatry clinic, eating disorders programs, Assertive Community Treatment teams, and psychotherapy.

Exposure to outpatient psychiatric practice can be more challenging to provide. An option for outpatient psychiatric treatment is to develop a student-facilitated outpatient psychiatry clinic supervised by a team of dedicated attending psychiatrists. This experience allows more active involvement by students in patient interviews under direct supervision.

"Enrichment learning activities" may be developed and required, often in coordination with community resources. Attendance at an Alcoholic Anonymous or Narcotics Anonymous meeting, a visit to a rehabilitation day program for patients with severe mental illness, or home visits with a community support worker may make memorable teaching experiences. These activities are best performed with close coordination of community resources and "debriefing" of the experiences.

Both selectives and enrichment activities are best offered after a related formal clerkship didactic (e.g., offer a selective half-day in geriatric psychiatry clinic after the geriatric psychiatry didactic) or with advance required readings or online modules. The benefits of enrichment must be weighed against the time and resources needed to provide a high-quality experience for students and the time that they spend away from their primary site.

### *MANAGING STUDENT CONCERNS*

Students present for their psychiatry clerkship with not only the typical anxiety they bring to other clerkships but also often with further concerns about interacting with patients with mental illnesses. Most will have had minimal contact with psychiatrists or psychiatric patients prior to medical school as opposed to other branches of medicine. Many come with preconceived biases that are best discussed openly at the start of the clerkship. Such ideas may include that psychiatric patients are chronically ill, that treatments are limited and ineffective, that prognoses are poor, that it will be difficult to connect with psychiatric patients, and that working in inpatient sites is highly stressful or dangerous.

The clerkship director's own real-world experience with patient care should clearly impart a sense of optimism to the students about psychiatric treatment. At orientation, an outline of a psychiatric assessment with the history of present illness, longitudinal psychiatric history, and a comprehensive psychiatric screen for comorbidity can give students a greater sense of confidence and a framework they can use immediately.

The role of primary care physicians, including internists, family practitioners, pediatricians, and obstetricians and gynecologists, in providing psychiatric assessment and first-line treatment should be reinforced.

Students should know that they are unlikely to "avoid" psychiatric patients no matter what specialty they choose and that treating such patients can be rewarding. If the clerkship director projects enthusiasm about the clinical mission and beneficial interactions of psychiatry with other disciplines, students will be more receptive.

Students are likely to encounter agitated or hostile patients. They should be instructed to remove themselves from situations in which they feel threatened or uncomfortable, interview high-risk patients in public areas, and report any verbal or physical threats from patients immediately to their site and clerkship directors. If clinical experiences trigger a strong or confusing emotional reaction for the student, a meeting with the clerkship director should occur.

## Teaching and Learning in the Clerkship

### *STUDENT ORIENTATION*

Large-group orientation on the first day of the clerkship and frequent, clear email communications from the clerkship coordinator are the best methods of setting and maintaining student expectations and responsibilities. The clerkship orientation is generally a half-day meeting on the first morning of the rotation that is attended by all students, the clerkship director, and the clerkship coordinator. Each site's unique features should be described, including information about site-specific orientation, parking and security access, expectations for hours of attendance, appropriate attire, patient care routine, electronic medical records, expectations for student documentation, and any required weekend or nighttime call or rounding. The process for unexpected and requested absences should be discussed. About 3 weeks prior to starting the clerkship, the coordinator should send all upcoming students the absence policy in writing. Any requirement for assigned makeup work for elective absences should be outlined.

Didactic schedules should be presented in writing at the orientation. Generally, attendance by students to clerkship didactics takes precedence over clinical duties. Students should be instructed what to do if an unusual clinical situation arises that would delay their participation. Expectations and timelines for written assignments, completion of patient logs, or individual reports and presentations should be provided in writing at orientation. A summary page may be created and placed in an orientation booklet with contact information and a list of the essential assignments, clinical references, and due dates. This document can serve as a reference for students throughout their rotation.

The clerkship orientation is the ideal opportunity to educate students about the elements and techniques of a standardized psychiatric assessment interview, including the mental status examination. Many will have had limited information or recollection about how to conduct a psychiatric assessment interview from their preclinical curriculum. Standardized psychiatric rating tools for students (e.g., Patient Health Questionnaire–9, the Mood Disorders Questionnaire, the Adult ADHD Self-Report Scale) should be provided to assist in patient assessments.

Opportunities for bidirectional feedback regarding student experiences should be made available during the clerkship. Group or individual "feedback meetings" with the clerkship director midway and at the end of the rotation should be supplemented by optional written feedback because students may have information that they feel more comfortable sharing in writing. Students should be instructed to contact the clerkship director immediately if their experiences diverge significantly from the expectations outlined at orientation.

Students are keenly interested in and motivated by the grading process of the clerkship. The grading protocol used by the clerkship should be described in explicit detail at the orientation and a written summary of the grading scheme should be provided. The grading system must remain unchanged throughout the academic year; modifications must be instituted at the start of the next academic year. See Chapter 10 for a more thorough discussion of evaluation strategies.

### *DIDACTICS*

Standard lectures typically cover the mental status examination, psychopharmacology, and common diagnoses and should both be clinically relevant and reinforce testable content seen on end-of-clerkship and the USMLE Step 2 examinations. A major difference at the clerkship level is the development of interpersonal and observational skills that generate clinical competence rather than declarative knowledge as experienced in the preclinical stage (McFarlane et al. 1989). Formal didactics provide better equivalence in knowledge if clinical sites are not uniform and ensures that the clerkship leadership and coordinator can "check in" with learners.

Half-days in the afternoon for didactics at a central site allow students to complete morning or rounding duties and then be free for didactic meetings. Didactic time may also introduce psychiatry students to interest groups or to faculty providing mentorship. The clerkship director should select teachers who enrich clinical material and link that material to practical diagnostics and clinical decision making in an active learning format. Junior faculty, interested residents, and fellows may be recruited to teach didactics. Individuals who are developmentally closer to medical students can often offer an instruction level more appropriate to their needs.

### *RESIDENTS AS TEACHERS*

LCME 9.1 requires residents who supervise or teach medical students to be familiar with the objectives of the clerkship and to be prepared for the responsibility of teaching and evaluating students. The clerkship director is responsible for providing the clerkship objectives to all residents who are involved with medical students. New residents should be provided interactive sessions on clinical teaching, coaching medical students, and giving productive formative and summative feedback. Program directors can use these non-bedside teaching sessions as part of resident evaluations and to fulfill ACGME milestones. Formal feedback from students can document the effectiveness of resident teaching.

## CONCLUSION

Designing a preclinical course in psychiatry has changed significantly over time, with widespread integration of basic sciences, doctoring principles, and interactive learning platforms. It is imperative that course directors use available guidelines and standards to implement engaging learning activities. Psychiatry clerkship directors should be astute clinicians who have a passion for teaching and enhancing the image of psychiatry within their institution. Psychiatry clerkships vary in length at different institutions but share the mandate to provide students a varied and rich clinical experience with engaged preceptors while ensuring equivalency between training sites.

Although there is reliance on traditional inpatient sites for training medical students, the thoughtful use of volunteer faculty, community resources, outpatient clinics, and specialty clinics can enhance a psychiatry clerkship experience. A thorough student orientation at the beginning of the rotation and an engaged and mature clerkship coordinator are important ingredients to clerkship success.

## — KEY POINTS —

- Course director duties include working with basic science faculty to design a behavioral science or psychiatry course with an understanding of curriculum reform and major trends in curricular development.

- A preclinical course should utilize major clinical diagnoses as a framework within the context of innovative teaching methods.
- The clerkship director must ensure that rotations fulfill the requirements of the Liaison Committee on Medical Education while taking into account the unique needs and demands of their own institutions.
- Optimal clerkship length and whether to combine the psychiatry clerkship with that of other specialties are sources of ongoing debate.
- Offering varied clinical experiences for students while attaining and ensuring equivalency between training sites is an important task of the clerkship director.
- Volunteer faculty and psychiatry residents are important members of the clinical teaching team and need support and mentorship.

# REFERENCES

Bobo W, Nevin R, Greene E, Lacy T: The effect of psychiatric third-year rotation setting on academic performance, student attitudes, and specialty choice. Acad Psychiatry 33:105–111, 2009

Brauer DG, Ferguson KJ: The integrated curriculum in medical education: AMEE Guide No. 96. Med Teach 37:312–322, 2015

Carney PA, Palmer RT, Fuqua Miller M, et al: Tools to assess behavioral and social science competencies in medical education: a systematic review. Acad Med 91:730–742, 2016

Clegg K: Combined clerkships. Paper presented at the annual meeting of the Association of Directors of Medical Student Education in Psychiatry, Jackson Hole, WY, June 2003

Cooke M, Irby DM, O'Brien BC: Educating physicians: a call for reform of medical school and residency. San Francisco, CA, Jossey-Bass, 2010

Harden RM: Approaches to curriculum planning. Med Educ 20:458–466, 1986

Harper BL, Roman BJB: The changing landscape of recruitment in psychiatry. Acad Psychiatry 41:221–225, 2017

Hawa R, Klapheke M, Liu H, et al: An innovative technology blueprint for medical education: association of directors of medical student education in psychiatry's clinical simulation initiative years 1–6. Acad Psychiatry 41:408–410, 2017

Institute of Medicine: Improving Medical Education: Enhancing the Behavioral and Social Science Content of Medical School Curricula. Washington, DC, National Academies Press, 2004

Iyer A: Why medical students should consider psychiatry. Op-Med, August 23, 2017. Available at: https://opmed.doximity.com/articles/why-medical-students-should-consider-psychiatry?_csrf_attempted=yes. Accessed January 18, 2020.

Klement BJ, Paulsen DF, Wineski LE: Clinical correlations as a tool in basic science medical education. J Med Educ Curric Dev 3:179–185, 2016
Kumar A, Kallen D, Mathew T: Volunteer faculty: what rewards or incentives do they prefer? Teach Learn Med 14:119–123, 2002
Liaison Committee on Medical Education: Functions and Structure of a Medical School: Standards for Accreditation of Medical Education Programs Leading to the MD Degree. Washington, DC, Association of American Medical Colleges, 2019. Available at: https://lcme.org/wp-content/uploads/filebase/standards/2020-21_Functions-and-Structure_2019-10-04.docx. Accessed January 18, 2020.
Markham B: Can a behavioral science course change medical students' attitudes? Acad Psychiatry 3:44–54, 1979
McFarlane AC, Goldney RD, Kalucy RS: A factor analytic study of clinical competence in undergraduate psychiatry. Med Educ 23:422–428, 1989
McGeehan J, English R, Shenberger K, et al: A community continuity programme: volunteer faculty mentors and continuity learning. Clin Teach 10:15–20, 2013
Niedermier J, Way D, Kasick D, Kuperschmidt R: Effect of curriculum change on exam performance in a 4-week psychiatry clerkship. Acad Psychiatry 34:216–219, 2010
Pangaro L, Bachicha J, Brodkey A, et al: Expectations of and for clerkship directors: a collaborative statement from the Alliance for Clinical Education. Teach Learn Med 15:217–222, 2003
Retamero C, Ramchandani D: Subspecialty exposure in psychiatry clerkship does not improve student performance in the subject examination. Acad Psychiatry 37:179–181, 2013
Roman B, Schatte D, Frank J, et al: The ADMSEP Milestones Project. Acad Psychiatry 40:314–316, 2016
Rosenthal R, Levine R, Carlson D, et al: The "shrinking" clerkship: characteristics and length of clerkships in psychiatry undergraduate education. Acad Psychiatry 29:47–51, 2005
Schwartzstein RM, Roberts DH: Saying goodbye to lectures in medical school—paradigm shift or passing fad? N Engl J Med 377:605–607, 2017
Starr SR, Agrwal N, Bryan MJ, et al: Science of health care delivery: an innovation in undergraduate medical education to meet society's needs. Mayo Clin Proc Innov Qual Outcomes 1:117–129, 2017

# CHAPTER 8

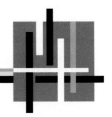

# SPECIAL CONSIDERATIONS IN MEDICAL STUDENT EDUCATION

Katharine J. Nelson, M.D.
Lora Wichser, M.D.

**Things** *are different now.* This chapter is informed by our personal experience mentoring and advising medical students and psychiatry residents over the past decade and provides a broad overview of some of the unprecedented issues now facing medical students and psychiatric trainees. As psychiatric educators and clinicians, it may be tempting at times to utter phrases such as

- "I would have never done that when I was a medical student."
- "What makes these residents think this is okay?"
- "When I was a trainee, I was responsible for much more."
- "Why are these learners so coddled? I never had a 'safe space'!"

The intent of this chapter is to illustrate the many ways in which the social, cultural, political, and health care system and accelerated technological changes have created a vastly different educational landscape. It is not accurate or effective to contrast one's own medical training with the experience of current medical students and trainees in psychiatry.

We use reflections and vignettes to illustrate concepts pertinent to contemporary psychiatric education. *Things are just different now.*

# INFORMATION OVERLOAD

The pace of technological change since the early 1990s, coupled with the ability to access information instantly, is unprecedented. Prior to the internet, medical learners relied on textbooks, slides, handouts, lectures, and chalk talks. This approach (rigorous and challenging in its own right) provided the basic and continuing education necessary to support medical practice. Individuals who learned in the prior model often marvel at the ready access to information provided by technological advancements: "If only I had had access to this kind of information when I was a medical student! These students are so lucky to be training in this era."

## Challenges Presented by Technology

This vast array of medical and scientific information of varying quality poses a serious challenge for emerging medical professionals. New medical trainees are often overwhelmed by the sheer quantity, availability, and variability of information. Medical educators sometimes lack the insight and skills to transition to teaching practices that account for this new reality. Well-meaning educators sometimes provide students with copious resources, such as links, articles, videos, or online modules. The trainees may experience this as overwhelming because there is no reasonable way to digest and assimilate such a large quantity of information. The stress of this excessive cognitive load impacts the well-being of medical trainees, who experience self-doubt and worry they will harm a future patient due to their inability to register vast quantities of detailed information (Young et al. 2014). Medical educators must therefore serve as curators of information and construct clear and basic conceptual learning frameworks to help students build the cognitive scaffolding related to a particular content area. Once this foundation is built, students may then obtain higher-level, more detailed information to further refine and elucidate their understanding of a particular topic (Ambrose et al. 2010; de Jong 2010; Halpern and Hakel 2003).

## The Myth of "Spoon-Feeding"

When educators receive feedback about information overload or student inquiries about which content will be tested, they often recoil and suggest that learners are asking to be "spoon-fed" information. This understandable yet judgmental reaction to learners' concerns may be based on self-referential thinking and recall about being held responsible for self-learning goals. Such thinking is misplaced in the context of the current volume of information. Trainees feel invalidated and marginalized when they hear the suggestion that they are not assuming personal responsibility for learning and thus may be conditioned to not disclose their concerns for fear of appearing "unprofessional" or "lazy" (Jauregui et al. 2020).

## Standardized Testing

Further complicating this issue is the fact that the U.S. Medical Licensing Examination (USMLE), Comprehensive Osteopathic Medical Licensing Examination of the United States (COMLEX-USA), and specialty board examinations require trainees to be held accountable for vast quantities of often-unpredictable information. The practice of using USMLE scores to filter residency applicants for competitive specialties adds to the mandate that students memorize as much information as possible to prepare for examinations or risk exclusion from a desired future specialty. In addition, emerging data suggest that this type of standardized testing may exhibit bias against learners who are from underprivileged or underrepresented backgrounds (Boatright et al. 2017). In response to advocacy aimed at decreasing unnecessary stress on medical students and steps to promote a more holistic and equitable residency selection process, the Federation of State Medical Boards and National Board of Medical Examiners announced that the USMLE Step 1 examination would transition to pass/fail (rather than numeric) scoring beginning January 1, 2022. The USMLE Step 2 clinical knowledge and Step 3 examinations will continue to be numerically scored. The National Board of Osteopathic Medical Examiners has stated that the COMLEX-USA Level 1 examination will continue to be numerically scored pending further study.

## Generational Divide and the Resilience Problem

Rapidly expanding technology and information contributes to an accelerating generational divide within medicine. These fast and frequent changes often mean that the expectations, needs, and perspectives for residents preparing to graduate differ even from those that were in place for their recently graduated contemporaries. Because of this, medical students may be inappropriately perceived as having limited frustration tolerance, irritability, impaired "resilience," and an unbecoming desire for comfort or "safety." This unfair emphasis on the students' level of resilience and safety is why we use this terminology carefully and use quotation marks to designate circumstances in which the terms are applied unfairly. Medical schools across the country have made efforts to improve the resilience of medical students. Many such efforts are well-founded when students bear the burden of unnecessary shame, embarrassment, depression, fatigue, or anxiety related to imposter syndrome or other impediments. Other attempts are unfounded and inappropriate because the problem is not resilience but that aspects of the medical training system produce cognitive overload well beyond reasonable limits. This severely impacts students. Educators must identify systems-based issues unnecessarily impacting students rather than place the responsibility on students to increase their "resilience" to better tolerate potentially harmful circumstances (Jauregui et al. 2020).

## Case Example: Bao

Bao is excited to begin his first rotation in psychiatry. One week before the rotation, Bao receives an email from the coordinator requesting that he complete required onboarding paperwork for his clinical site. He must apply for a badge that will allow him access to the inpatient unit, create an account with the hospital credentialing system, and attest that he will follow required privacy practices, complete online modules related to the importance of handwashing, and review the quality aims of the hospital system. He must affirm his commitment not to engage in sexual harassment or maltreatment and complete an additional module screening him for well-being related issues, such as depression, burnout, or suicide. He must create an account and register his credit card with the hospital parking services to park his car. He must download a third-party mobile application to complete evaluations on his cell phone. Bao is asked to set up his account and password with the hospital's electronic medical record and complete the required training modules. He is provided a link to a website where he is asked to create an account and place a deposit on the pager that is required for the clerkship. Another link is provided to complete an online poll for required call activities. Failure to complete these activities is considered "out of compliance" and will be referred to the Peer Review Committee of the medical school. Bao must complete similar activities every 4 weeks prior to starting rotations.

Midway through the rotation, he receives an email stating that he has failed to attest within the online learning management system that he requested and received verbal feedback from his supervisor. As a result, two points will be deducted from his overall points due to lack of professionalism. Bao feels demoralized and somewhat resentful because he believes this is unfair. Bao urgently searches his email and locates a communication from the course director sent 2 weeks earlier describing the requirement that midrotation feedback be obtained and an attestation be completed on the online learning management system. Bao feels inept and irresponsible for missing the email and resolves to monitor for similar communications in the future. He is frustrated by the multiple systems requirements he is expected to complete for each rotation. He had considered a career in psychiatry but now wonders if his final grade will allow this.

### Questions for Reflection

1. What themes did you notice about Bao's required preparation for his rotation?
2. Are the expectations similar to when you completed medical student rotations?
3. What consequences exist for Bao losing points for lack of "professionalism"?

# PSYCHOLOGICAL THREATS AND ESTABLISHING SAFETY

In addition to the cognitive overload associated with the digital age, students and medical trainees also experience stress related to psychosocial aspects of medical training.

## Representation Matters

A diverse medical workforce will more effectively serve the public. The Accreditation Council for Graduate Medical Education (ACGME; 2018) has acknowledged this and incorporated requirements promoting diversity (see Chapter 6). Proactively increasing diversity and inclusion requires taking steps to transform our educational and clinical learning environments to minimize harms to students from underrepresented groups. Of particular importance is advancing the visible representation of racial, ethnic, disabled, religious, gender, sexual orientation, and other marginalized identities in leadership in academic medicine (Dasgupta and Greenwald 2001; Martell 1991; Walton and Cohen 2007, 2011).

## Imposter Syndrome

Homogeneous leadership results in pervasive invalidation for students from underrepresented communities and constitutes a form of minority stress (Dyrbye et al. 2006; Sitkin and Pachankis 2016). Such trainees routinely describe feeling like imposters in the classroom or clinical learning environment (Villwock et al. 2016) and making automatic assumptions such as "I don't belong here," "I was let in by mistake," "Maybe I was only admitted because the medical school needed more people of color to meet a quota," or "Do I really have the credentials and experience to succeed in medicine?"

A common early medical school course is anatomy lab—an experience that those who are underrepresented in medicine often arrive to ill prepared compared with peers whose physician family members have prepared them with their personal experiences. Emotional responses to seeing a human cadaver also differ based on cultural upbringing, further isolating students who do not share the more prevalent cultural response to discomfort or disgust: "My religion highly values the sanctity of the body. To cut someone's dead body feels deeply wrong. It takes all of my strength of will to make it through anatomy lab, let alone trying to learn anything. Praying before and after would help me feel better—but no one else is doing this. What's wrong with me?" This incongruence between a student's internal experience and what is perceived to be the experience of others results in a questioning of the legitimacy of one's own internal experiences. This may be particularly pronounced for trainees who have lived or had previous training in an international setting.

## "Practice on Each Other"

Another contributor to psychological distress in the training environment is the routine practice of encouraging students to practice on their classmates to learn medical examination skills. Students whose cultural observances require covering of the body may object to uncovering parts of their body for this purpose. Students who have experienced trauma also may have difficulty with physical contact and may not wish to discuss this openly. Trainees with varying body shapes and sizes may experience self-consciousness or shame related to their belief that others will perceive them as "unhealthy" or having a "nonpreferred physique" for a health care professional (Dasgupta and Greenwald 2001; Martell 1991; Walton and Cohen 2007, 2011).

### Case Example: Angelita

Angelita has experienced the first year of medical school to be extremely stressful given the academic demands and the social milieu and hierarchy. Angelita identifies with a societal expectation that women must remove hair from their feet and legs as a part of routine grooming. Due to exhaustion and lack of time, Angelita has not adhered to this societal expectation and instead has chosen to wear clothing that covers her legs.

During the small group for the foot and ankle examination learning session, the preceptor directs the students to roll up their pant legs and remove socks and shoes to practice examinations on one another. Angelita is embarrassed for what she perceives is a lack of appropriate grooming. She worries she will disgust her group and feels she must apologize to her preceptor and the other group members. At the end of the learning session, Angelita feels anxious and exhausted and has learned little.

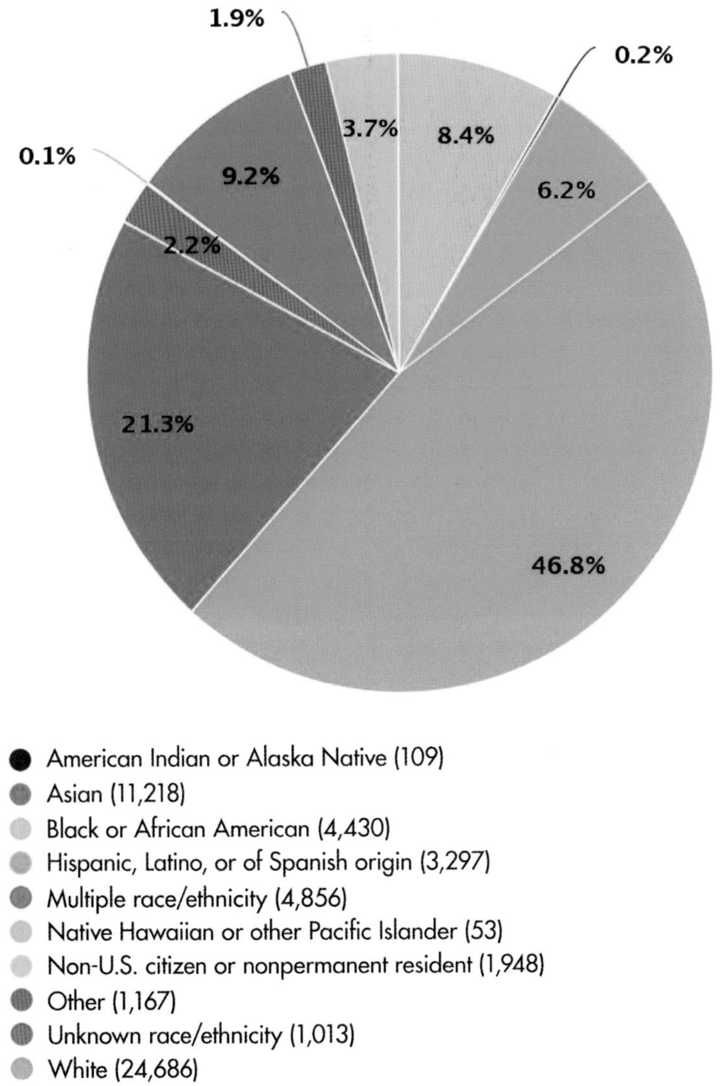


**PLATE 1. Percentage of applicants to U.S. medical schools by race/ethnicity (alone), academic year 2018–2019.**

Race/Ethnicity "alone" indicates that an individual is reported in only one race/ethnicity category. The "Multiple race/ethnicity" category includes individuals who selected more than one race/ethnicity response. The "Non-U.S. citizen or nonpermanent resident" category may include individuals with unknown citizenship.

*Source.* Association of American Medical Colleges (2020a).

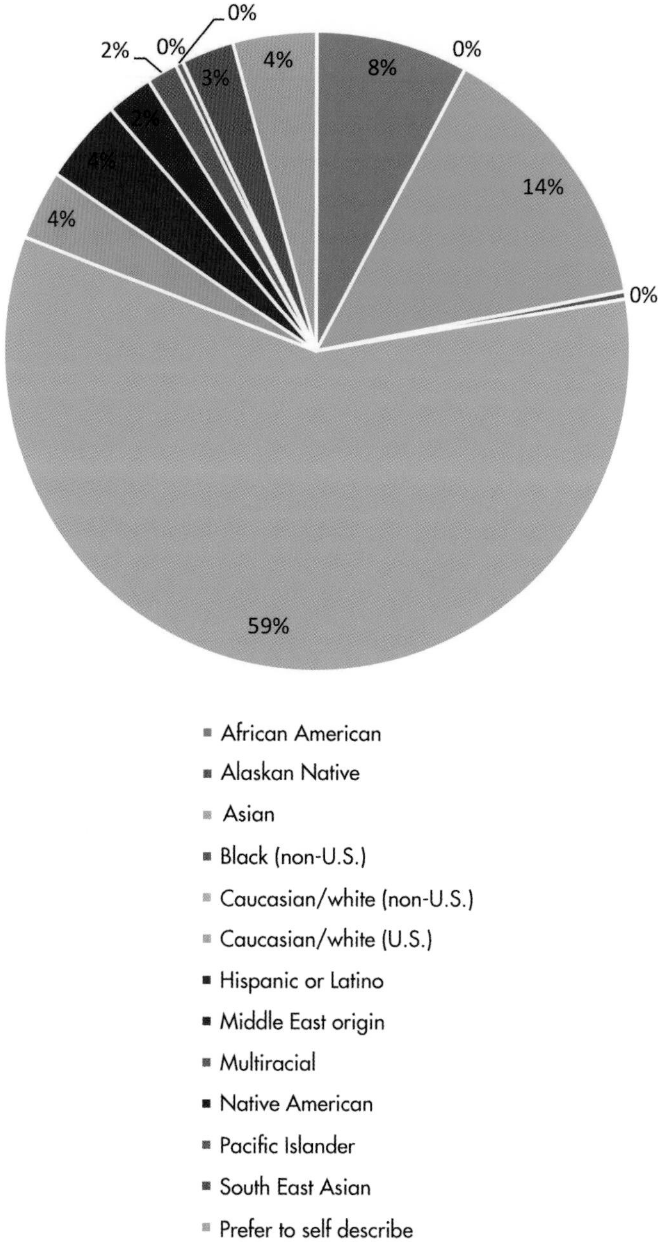


**PLATE 2. American Association of Directors of Psychiatric Residency Training survey on diversity—membership: Which race/ethnicity best describes you?**
*Source.* Adams 2019.

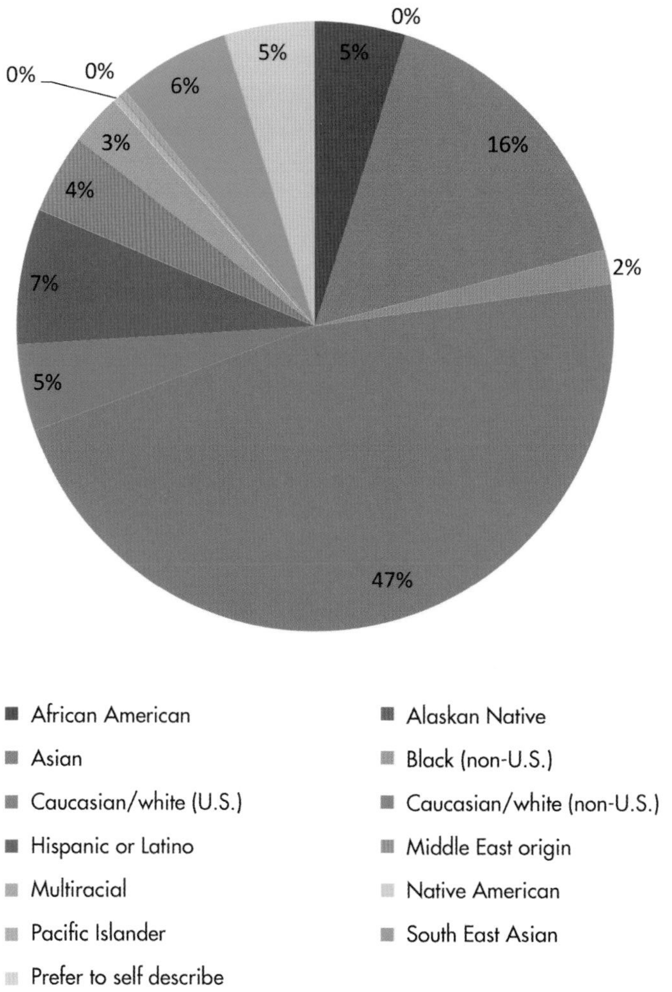


**PLATE 3. American Association of Directors of Psychiatric Residency Training survey on diversity—trainees: Which race/ethnicity best describes you?**
*Source.* Adams 2019.

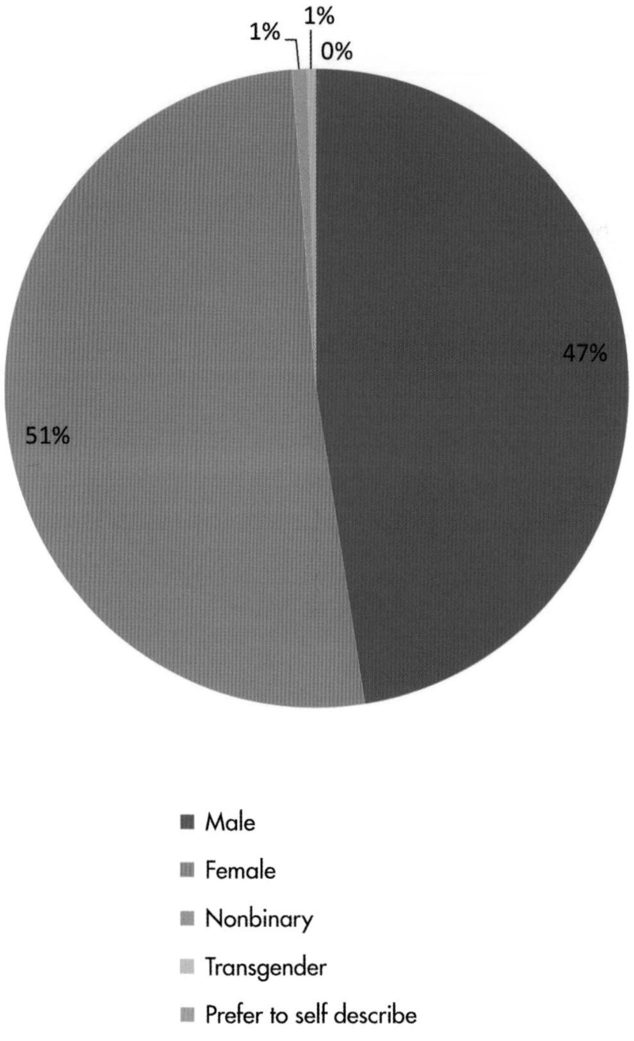


**PLATE 4. American Association of Directors of Psychiatric Residency Training survey on diversity—trainees: What is your gender identity?**
*Source.* Adams 2019.

Angelita feels like an imposter because the other members of the small group seemed comfortable.

### Questions for Reflection

1. What themes did you notice about Angelita's experience in small group?
2. Were expectations similar when you completed physical examination training?
3. What are the consequences of peer physical examinations for a student?

## Illness Anxiety

As students learn about pathological states, they naturally scan for salience and the applicability of this new knowledge to themselves or to people in their family. It is not uncommon for students to approach a lecturer and disclose a belief that they might have the diagnosis discussed in class. Students may even obtain screening to assess for the disorder. This anxiety is complicated by the fact that medical students are not exempt from experiencing serious medical conditions during training.

### Case Example: Terry

Terry is a second-year medical student who always had access to regular medical care but has never experienced a major illness. During the head and neck lecture, the presenter encourages the students to palpate their neck to identify anatomical landmarks. Terry feels a firm fixed lump on the right side of their neck behind their jaw and ear. They hear the lecturer say, "A unilateral neck mass is cancer until proven otherwise."

Terry is immediately concerned and assumes that they have neck cancer. Terry makes an appointment with a general surgeon to examine their neck. They are scheduled for an evaluation in 2 weeks, and while waiting, they frequently palpate their neck and ask others to do likewise. They cannot sleep and wake in the middle of night to feel the lump. They are having difficulty studying for midterm examinations. Finally, they briefly meet with a general surgeon who palpates their neck and determines that the lump likely represents a tense muscle or a bony protrusion. Terry is surprised that they were not being referred for biopsy or imaging. They have difficulty reconciling the outcome of the assessment with what they have learned in the classroom.

### Questions for Reflection

1. What themes did you notice about Terry's learning new medical information and applying this information to themself?
2. What has been your experience with illness anxiety in your medical training?

3. What consequences exist for Terry in learning and applying new information to their personal health?

# MANAGING IMPEDIMENTS TO SURVIVAL AND ACHIEVEMENT

In this section we explore the challenges trainees may encounter that impact their choices and behavior as they seek to overcome barriers to achievement.

## "Professionalism"

The term *professionalism* has long been used in medical training to describe the essential features of medical practice. We once again place a word in quotation marks to reference circumstances in which this term is inappropriately applied. Students and trainees are routinely assessed for their degree of professionalism. Sometimes, the measure of professionalism is observable behavior, such as timeliness. However, this term has been used to capture intangible aspects about trainee behavior in the clinical training environment, so "professionalism" may inappropriately identify students who fail to behave in a manner that affirms the evaluators' perception of an ideal physician. Such perceptions of "professionalism" are often overly informed by self-reference and the evaluators' sociocultural lens.

One primary example may be found in the residency interview process. Interview processes for residency by which interviewers work to determine whether a student will "fit in" are a superficial means of hiring that risk propagating stereotypes and enacting overt and implicit biases (Shappell and Schnapp 2019). Students who do not fit the expected "mold" may experience a sense of helplessness if held to a standard that they do not fully understand and are not empowered to meet (Lee 2017).

### Case Example: Dustin

Dustin is a third-year medical student raised in a single-parent lower socioeconomic household. His mother held a regular job as a waitress working the 4 P.M.–1 A.M. shift weeknights and one weekend day. Because his mother usually slept until 9 A.M., Dustin grew up sleeping later, quietly going about his day until his mother awoke and took him to school. He is a fast learner, very personable, and received encouragement and support in elementary and high school to achieve academically.

Dustin enjoyed his anesthesiology rotation and thought this might be a good career choice. He was shocked to see a grade of "satisfactory" rather than "excellent" or "honors" on his evaluation. The narrative comments said he had demonstrated a notable lack of professionalism throughout the rotation by arriving 5–10 minutes late every morning. Dustin thought the team understood that he was taking public transportation and that his arrival time would be somewhat variable. He had believed that his arrival time was generally acceptable. Nobody told him that arriving 10 minutes past the published start time would be perceived as unprofessional. He felt helpless to correct his grade and wondered if he owed team members and supervisors an apology. He felt angry and resentful that he would be held to an inflexible or unachievable standard. On his previous rotation his preceptor had indicated that it was acceptable for his arrival to be variable. Dustin had received the grade of "excellent" for this rotation.

Although Dustin enjoyed anesthesiology, he eliminated this profession as a career choice because he believed that he could no longer be competitive.

### Questions for Reflection

1. What themes did you notice about Dustin's meeting expectations for professional behavior?
2. What was your experience with meeting expectations for professionalism in your medical training?
3. What are the consequences for Dustin's growth and development arising from this evaluation and feedback?

## Perfectionism

As psychiatric education works to improve the integrity and accuracy of evaluation, best practices suggest more frequent, lower-stakes opportunities for evaluation, with appropriate coaching and feedback (Dunlosky et al. 2013; Halpern and Hakel 2003; Larsen et al. 2009; Roediger et al. 2011; Tanner 2013). Whereas high-stakes evaluations are unfair, unreliable, and clearly contribute to stress, more frequent evaluations contribute to the sense that a student is being constantly evaluated and thus not permitted to have a "bad" day. This pressure to perform may result in students going to extraordinary lengths to appear competent and even "perfect." Students may suppress or deny their basic needs, including using the bathroom, accessing water and food, sleeping, or lactating.

### Case Example: Carmen

Carmen is a fourth-year medical student on an away rotation in psychiatry where she hopes to achieve a residency position. She feels an intense desire to impress everyone on the treatment team. She carries a large number of patients and volunteers to assist with admissions. She skips breakfast and lunch because she does not want to sacrifice time that could be spent providing patient care and completing documentation, often eating a protein bar in the hallway while walking to conferences, hoping this will be sufficient nutrition for the day. At the end of a long day, while walking out to the parking ramp, she notices that she urgently needs to urinate. She is exhausted and decides to wait until she arrives home. On her drive home, she loses control of her bladder. She is ashamed, embarrassed, and disgusted. She cries the rest of the way home and questions whether she is truly prepared to begin residency.

### Questions for Reflection

1. What themes did you notice about Carmen's experience with meeting expectations for this high-stakes period of evaluation?
2. What has been your experience with being evaluated in a high-stakes environment in the context of your medical training?
3. What are the consequences for Carmen's professional identity arising from this incident?

## Family Planning, Fertility, Parenting, and Caregiving

Trainee fertility and family planning is a serious matter that is infrequently explored or discussed, despite the fact that trainees of all genders often train at an age when developing family relationships and reproduction are salient goals. This urgency is heightened as they learn about periods of peak fertility and the potential health risks and outcomes associated with pregnancy at later ages. Adoption or pursuing surrogacy are also more difficult as the trainee ages. Trainees may be exploring and understanding sexual or gender identity, considering a long-term relationship's status, or pursuing a new relationship. People who choose to have children during medical school or residency may be viewed as "unprofessional" by some who believe it places personal goals above the health of patients or the community. To combat the threat of this stereotype, physician parents may feel both internal and external pressure to overachieve in order to prove their commitment to the profession.

Trainees who choose to delay family expansion face the pressure and potential expense of harvesting eggs or storing sperm to increase the odds of a later healthy pregnancy. Trainees who desire partners may feel conflicted because medical education often interferes with normal social activities that help identify a partner. The culture of medicine has historically invalidated partnership, family planning, or fertility concerns as being self-focused or even "selfish." Trainees may also be required to provide care for a family member or a loved one with an illness. Such needs may constitute an unmanageable circumstance in which demands far outpace resources (Stentz et al. 2016).

## Bias, Harassment, and Discrimination

Students may face sexual harassment, racism, nationalism, homophobia, transphobia, ableism, or other forms of discrimination and bias while in training. Given power imbalances, trainees often feel pressed to overlook, ignore, or deny the impact of such experiences. Trainees identifying as *advocates* are often confused when their patients or fellow team members have differing political views and values. Students benefit from validation of internal stress, distress, or conflict related to these experiences. Most institutions mandate the reporting of harassment. Trainees often feel conflicted about reporting, fearing retribution or poor evaluations. It is the responsibility of institutions and those in authority to build trustworthy systems and respond appropriately and confidentially when harassment is reported (Brill 2016).

## Personal Finances

Another source of substantial stress for medical students is finances. Historically, many medical trainees have been raised in privileged backgrounds with family financial support. As medical schools have appropriately taken steps to include more students from underprivileged backgrounds, the ancillary costs of medical school take a serious toll, underestimated by medical education leaders and educators.

### Case Example: Lamar

Lamar is second-year medical student. He did not do as well on his USMLE Step 1 standardized examination as he hoped, so he feels enormous pressure to sufficiently prepare for the USMLE Step 2 examination. His adviser recommends that he attend a commercial test preparation course that costs $2,500. Lamar supports himself with loans and has no savings or family members to financially contribute. He decides to obtain a part-time job to defray the cost of the course at the risk of further lessening his time for study.

### Questions for Reflection

1. What themes did you notice about Lamar's experience with financial stress?
2. What has been your experience with financial stress during medical training?
3. What are the consequences for Lamar in both his personal and professional life?

## PRIOR EXPERIENCES AS HEALTH CARE RECIPIENTS

Students who have prior personal experiences as health care recipients may experience stress as they are reminded about traumatic health care experiences. This is particularly true in psychiatry if students or their loved ones have received mental health treatment (Brenner et al. 2018). Students may underestimate the impact of such experiences. The stress of such events may be mitigated somewhat with anticipatory guidance to students and normalization of the phenomena during orientation, as well as encouragement to reach out to their support system.

All health care professionals and trainees are at risk of verbal or physical assault in the clinical learning environment. Serious events of this nature are a known risk; students are particularly vulnerable in that they may experience pressure to behave as though these assaults are not associated with significant personal impact. Students may feel a responsibility to "bounce back" from such events to reflect strength in the face of adversity. This compartmentalization may serve short-term goals at the expense of long-term mental health.

### Case Example: Lee

Lee is a 25-year-old medical student in their third year of training. While on clinical rotations, Lee has often heard patients described as "lifelong depressives" and "essentially unfixable." Lee has had episodes of depression since childhood and does not identify as a person who needs to be "fixed." Prior to this, Lee felt they got along well with other members of the team and felt a sense of belonging. Now, they feel distant from the team and wonders if this will negatively affect their evaluation. When feeling down, Lee wonders if indeed they are broken and "unfixable" and wonders if medicine really is the right field for them.

### Questions for Reflection

1. What themes did you notice about Lee's experience?
2. What has been your experience with lived illness during your medical training?
3. What are the consequences for Lee in both their personal and professional life?

## TO DISCLOSE OR NOT TO DISCLOSE?

Trainees who have psychiatric conditions that predate medical school often face enormous internal conflict about whether to disclose this condition to advisors, teachers, administrators, or program directors. Advisors are often also potential employers; dual roles of advisor and future program director may result in substantial fear of bias or discrimination. Data suggest that fear about potential discrimination for psychiatric conditions is well founded. Pheister et al. (2019) conducted a study and determined that the disclosure of a mental illness by medical students in their residency application decreased their chances of being invited for an interview and lowered their overall ranking for a residency position.

Students therefore experience conflict about disclosing the presence of a psychiatric condition in themselves or their close family members when writing the personal statement for residency applications. This fear is often compounded by state licensing boards that require information about the presence of psychiatric conditions or past psychiatric treatment. Students fear barriers in obtaining disability and life insurance or limited employment opportunities. Trainees who have conditions that necessitate learning and test-taking accommodations often face repeated shame in disclosing this fact.

## SUICIDE

Emerging literature demonstrates that physician trainees have a risk of suicide that is higher than the general population (Goldman et al. 2015). Death of a student or trainee represents the worst possible outcome in the context of medical education. It is incumbent upon the medical profession and those in leadership to enact clear and active strategies to mitigate the risk of trainees and practitioners dying from suicide. Chapter 3 reviews this issue in more detail.

## CONNECTEDNESS

An emerging theme in conversations across the psychiatric education continuum is the desire for trainees to experience a sense of connection with their internal values, their mission, and each other. Cognitive, psychological, and circumstantial stress may be buffered through a strong sense of community. Trainees may use social media in creative ways to establish cohorts, study groups, and special interest groups.

## CONCLUSION

Although this is not an exhaustive review of the multiple factors impacting psychiatric education, the special considerations we describe in this chapter are meant to challenge some of the automatic assumptions that may serve as a barrier to understanding the point of view of students, residents, and fellows. The educational landscape has been transformed to a point at which the educational setting is somewhat unrecognizable. Most importantly, please remember: *Things are just different now.*

## — KEY POINTS —

- Medical student and psychiatric trainees are facing unprecedented issues pertaining to the social, cultural, political, and health care systems and technological environment that have resulted in a vastly different educational landscape.
- The wide array of medical and scientific information of varying quality poses a serious challenge for emerging medical professionals and may result in cognitive overload due to the sheer quantity, availability, and variability of the information.
- Students and psychiatric trainees experience stress related to the psychosocial aspects of medical training, including consequences related to the lack of diverse representation across all levels of leadership, "imposter syndrome," illness anxiety, and microaggressions that detract from inclusion and psychological safety.
- Contextual impediments to survival and achievement for psychiatric trainees include financial challenges, perfectionism, family planning, fertility, parenting, caregiving, and consequences of bias, harassment, and discrimination.
- It is incumbent on the medical profession and those in leadership to enact clear and active strategies to mitigate the risk of trainees and practitioners dying from suicide, which represents the worst possible outcome in the context of medical education.

# REFERENCES

Accreditation Council for Graduate Medical Education: ACGME Common Program Requirements (Residency). Chicago, IL, Accreditation Council on Graduate Medical Education, 2018. Available at: https://www.acgme.org/Portals/0/PFAssets/ProgramRequirements/CPRResidency2019.pdf. Accessed November 11, 2020.

Ambrose SA, Bridges MW, DiPietro M, et al: How Learning Works: Seven Research-Based Principles for Smart Teaching. Hoboken, NJ, John Wiley and Sons, 2010

Boatright D, Ross D, O'Connor P, et al: Racial disparities in medical student membership in the Alpha Omega Alpha Honor Society. JAMA Intern Med 177(5):659–665, 2017

Brenner AM, Balon R, Guerrero AP, et al: Training as a psychiatrist when having a psychiatric illness. Acad Psychiatry 42(5):592–597, 2018
Brill D: Medical students stand up to sexual harassment. BMJ 354:i4430, 2016
Dasgupta N, Greenwald AG: On the malleability of automatic attitudes: combating automatic prejudice with images of admired and disliked individuals. J Pers Soc Psychol 81(5):800–814, 2001
de Jong T: Cognitive load theory, educational research, and instructional design: some food for thought. Instructional Science 38(2):105–134, 2010
Dunlosky J, Rawson KA, Marsh EJ, et al: Improving students' learning with effective learning techniques: promising directions from cognitive and educational psychology. Psychol Sci Public Interest 14(1):4–58, 2013
Dyrbye LN, Thomas MR, Huschka MM, et al: A multicenter study of burnout, depression, and quality of life in minority and nonminority US medical students. Mayo Clin Proc 81(11):1435–1442, 2006
Goldman ML, Shah RN, Bernstein CA, et al: Depression and suicide among physician trainees: recommendations for a national response. JAMA Psychiatry 72(5):411–412, 2015
Halpern DF, Hakel MD: Applying the science of learning to the university and beyond: teaching for long-term retention and transfer. Change: The Magazine of Higher Learning 35(4):36–41, 2003
Jauregui J, Watsjold B, Welsh L, et al: Generational 'othering': the myth of the Millennial learner. Med Educ 54(1):60–65, 2020
Larsen DP, Butler AC, Roediger III HL: Repeated testing improves long-term retention relative to repeated study: a randomized controlled trial. Med Educ 43(12):1174–1181, 2009
Lee JH: The weaponization of medical professionalism. Acad Med 92(5):579–580, 2017
Martell RF: Sex bias at work: the effects of attentional and memory demands on performance ratings of men and women. J Appl Soc Psychol 21(23):1939–1960, 1991
Pheister MA, Wrzosek M, Peters R: Illness disclosure in residency applications. Poster presented at the 48th Annual American Association of Directors of Psychiatric Residency Training, San Diego, CA, March 2, 2019
Roediger HL, Agarwal PK, McDaniel MA, McDermott KB: Test-enhanced learning in the classroom: long-term improvements from quizzing. J Exp Psychol Appl 17(4):382–395, 2011
Shappell E, Schnapp B: The F word: how "fit" threatens the validity of resident recruitment. J Grad Med Educ 11(6):635–636, 2019
Sitkin NA, Pachankis JE: Specialty choice among sexual and gender minorities in medicine: the role of specialty prestige, perceived inclusion, and medical school climate. LGBT Health 3(6):451–460, 2016
Stentz NC, Griffith KA, Perkins E, et al: Fertility and childbearing among American female physicians. J Womens Health 25(10):1059–1065, 2016
Tanner KD: Structure matters: twenty-one teaching strategies to promote student engagement and cultivate classroom equity. CBE Life Sci Educ 12(3):322–331, 2013
Villwock JA, Sobin LB, Koester LA: Impostor syndrome and burnout among American medical students: a pilot study. Int J Med Educ 7:364–369, 2016

Walton GM, Cohen GL: A question of belonging: race, social fit, and achievement. J Pers Soc Psychol 92(1):82–96, 2007

Walton GM, Cohen GL: A brief social-belonging intervention improves academic and health outcomes of minority students. Science 331(6023):1447–1451, 2011

Young JQ, Van Merrienboer J, Durning S, Ten Cate O: Cognitive load theory: implications for medical education: AMEE Guide No. 86. Med Teach 36(5):371–384, 2014

## CHAPTER 9

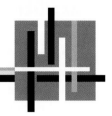

# RESIDENCY RECRUITMENT AND STUDENT ADVISING

Jessica Kovach, M.D.
John Spollen, M.D.
Lia A. Thomas, M.D.

**Recruitment** is an exciting but very busy time of the year for program directors. Successful recruiting is often key to the program director's performance evaluation and important for building the future of the program. Because recruitment trends vary from year to year, directors should pay attention to resources such as the American Association of Directors of Psychiatric Residency Training (AADPRT) listserv. We have divided this chapter into two sections: "Residency Recruitment" describes the basics of recruitment for program directors, and "Student Advising" provides information for those who advise students in choosing a specialty and applying to psychiatry residencies. Because program directors frequently work with medical students, they must keep the inherent conflicts of interest in mind when working with students who are also potential applicants.

# RESIDENCY RECRUITMENT

## Setting the Stage

We strongly recommend that programs establish recruitment goals and a plan to achieve those goals well in advance of recruitment season. Ideally, this should be completed in March or April, shortly after Match day. Establishing recruitment goals is best done by committee or departmental discussion. If your program has a diversity advisory committee, it should be part of this process. Although every program wants to recruit the "best" applicants, your committee should consider the experiences, attributes, and metrics that define the best applicant for *your* unique program. The definition of a successful resident in your program should align with your programmatic mission. Consider who has done well historically in your program and who has not. What attributes make a resident more likely to succeed in your program?

Once you have defined your program's "best" applicant, examine your online presence and consider whether the program's online presence is likely to attract applicants who will be the best fit. A program's online presence is one of the most important sources of information used by applicants to determine whether to apply. The online presence of which program directors have the most control is usually the program's website, which is one of the best opportunities to highlight program priorities, personality, and strengths. The website should contain clear information about the program's mission and distinguishing features. Examples of highlighted areas may include well-being, diversity, or a particular patient population. Applicants are likely to view the overall attention to detail and quality of a website as reflective of the quality of the program. Websites should be easy to navigate and visually attractive. Many academic centers have centralized advertising and information technology departments that should be utilized to help programs develop and maintain high-quality websites. Frequently, websites include a welcome letter from the program director followed by sections on current residents (including what medical schools the residents attended), the clinical program, didactic program, and alumni accomplishments. Other highlights may include resident scholarly or research accomplishments, information about local lifestyle and quality of life, and employee benefits. Applicants prefer that websites clearly state application requirements, including minimum or desired board scores.

An additional site is the Fellowship and Residency Electronic Interactive Database (FREIDA), provided by the Association of American Medical Colleges (AAMC), in which programs provide the program data available to applicants. You should complete FREIDA and utilize it in addition to other sites provided by reliable organizations. At the time of this writing, the AAMC is testing Residency Explorer, a tool for applicants to input their own data and compare it with matched residents in a given program. This tool is likely to be widely used in the future to help students navigate and select suitable residencies for which to apply. The "Student Advising" section later in the chapter further describes Residency Explorer.

A program's external image on third-party and crowd-sourcing sites is more difficult to influence. However, programs should be aware of these online data. Some sites allow programs to provide or edit information, whereas others do not. Awareness of online information about your program allows you to address misconceptions at the time of the interview or on your own website.

## Screening and Invitation to Interview

The Electronic Residency Application Service (ERAS) typically opens for program directors to view applications on September 15. Medical Student Performance Evaluation (MSPE; sometimes called "dean's letters") are available October 1. Currently, the average number of applications per psychiatry program is more than 1,000 (National Resident Matching Program 2019). Given this large volume of applications, well-organized screening strategies are important. One consideration is who will complete your screening: the program administrator/coordinator, associate program directors, chief residents, faculty committee, or just the program director? The time available will dictate how to best use such resources.

Methods used by programs vary from one person skimming through hundreds of applications and making quick "yes or no" determinations to complex ranking formulations that give weight to various application factors. Familiarize yourself with the sorting and filtering functions of ERAS. Items that are easy to sort and filter are often categorical or numerical. Examples include the presence or absence of a criminal record or the length of time since medical school graduation. More difficult items to sort or filter include qualitative items, such as geographical ties to a particular area or the depth and quality of volunteer experiences. Some programs send secondary applications to try to gauge applicant interest, but anecdotal reports about the usefulness of this practice are conflicting.

Your programmatic mission and a discussion of what type of applicants you want to recruit will help you to decide whom to invite to interview. Consider whether you can identify factors that will help you determine whether an applicant will want to attend or succeed in your program. To our knowledge, only one study evaluated the predictive value of application components in psychiatry (Brenner et al. 2010) by correlating any negative MSPE comments with future problems in residency. In other specialties, U.S. Medical Licensing Examination (USMLE) scores have been found to correlate with in-service examination scores and performance on specialty licensing board examinations (Boyse et al. 2002; Hartman et al. 2019; Raman et al. 2016; Stohl et al. 2010; Zuckerman et al. 2018). However, most studies fail to demonstrate correlation between USMLE scores and overall resident success or nonnumeric markers of resident success (Boyse et al. 2002; Hartman et al. 2019; Stohl et al. 2010; Zuckerman et al. 2018). Professionalism concerns in medical school have been correlated to future disciplinary action by medical boards (Papadakis et al. 2005).

Screening methods that view numerical data as one part of a holistic view of applicant attributes and strengths are more time intensive but possibly more equitable and successful. The AAMC describes a formal holistic review process as "mission-aligned admissions or selection processes that consider a broad range of factors—experiences, attributes, and academic metrics—when reviewing applications," and a full description of the process can be found on the AAMC website (Association of American Medical Colleges 2020b). Holistic review has been studied in the medical school admission process and found to be successful (Taylor et al. 2016). However, studies of holistic review in graduate medical education are limited to one paper describing an increase in applicants in one internal medicine program from groups who are underrepresented in medicine following implementation of a holistic review process (Aibana et al. 2019). See Chapter 6 for a further discussion of holistic review.

Programs must be conscious of the stress that scheduling interviews places on applicants. Applicants must juggle attendance at rotations, complex travel schedules, and travel expenses (not an inconsiderable concern for most medical students) when accepting interview invitations. Applicants generally appreciate flexibility in scheduling. Because some programs offer more interviews than they actually have available, applicants may feel pressured to check their email frequently and accept offers instantly. We discourage offering more interviews at any one time than the program has schedule slots available in order to minimize such stress.

After an applicant schedules an interview, most programs email information about the interview day, including the time, location, and anticipated interview schedule or length. Whenever possible, applicants prefer to receive a full detailed schedule, including the names of their interviewers. Usually programs provide travel information, such as suggested accommodations for out-of-town applicants, and ask in advance for dietary restrictions or other necessary accommodations for the interview day. Some programs offer other opportunities to personalize an interview day, such as identifying an applicant's preference to speak with a faculty or resident member who has particular expertise or with a faculty or resident member who identifies with a particular minority status or background.

Program directors also have reported receiving large numbers of personalized applicant emails during interview season. Program director attitudes about these emails vary. Some use them as an additional means to determine whether an applicant is interested in their program or will provide detailed answers to inquiries, whereas others prefer to use only ERAS applications and will disregard applicant emails. Some program directors welcome emails from faculty at other institutions recommending individual applicants, whereas others may not. Lack of standardization about this practice also puts stress on applicants who are often unclear as to how the program will regard them for sending or not sending such emails.

## The Interview Day

The interview day is the best opportunity for applicants and programs to evaluate each other. The mutual nature of this evaluation should be at the front of your mind as you plan the day. Remember that applicants will likely pay attention to how well the day is structured, how much time the program director and chair spend with them, and how much time they have with residents without faculty present. Most interview days start with an overall presentation about the school and the residency program, usually followed by a combination of individual interviews and tours.

Programs schedule between two and nine 15- to 45-minute individual interviews with faculty, residents, or a combination. Anecdotal feedback from students indicates that more than four or five interviews is exhausting and somewhat repetitive. Interview styles vary; some programs leave interviews unstructured or merely suggest interviewer questions, whereas others use very structured behavioral interviewing techniques. We strongly suggest that program directors hold a session in advance to educate interviewers about the program's interview expectations, Match policies, and any questions that must be avoided because of federal laws and Match restrictions. Written materials provided to the interviewers should include the most recent guidelines published by the National Residency Matching Program (NRMP). Generally, interviewers must provide some sort of structured feedback or numerical scoring of the applicant following the interview; examples of areas to score might include interpersonal skills, academic achievement, leadership skills, and psychological mindedness. Some programs give the applicants' entire ERAS application to interviewers in advance, whereas others choose to hold back certain areas such as USMLE scores to avoid bias or overemphasis on particular metrics.

Residents generally lead tours of the program and generally appreciate having a list of suggested tour stops such as the call room, cafeteria, library, and clinical areas. Resident tour guides also must often evaluate how the applicants behave in a group setting. Lunch is generally a good time for applicants to spend with residents without faculty present and can also be a chance to showcase some of the area's culinary culture. Be sure to accommodate dietary restrictions in advance.

## After the Interview

NRMP policies forbid programs from requiring communication with applicants after the interview day concludes. However, many applicants will send thank you notes to programs and interviewers. In recent years, fewer applicants have requested "second look" visits. Programs are forbidden from requiring a "second look" but are allowed to offer applicants the opportunity to return (e.g., to attend resident didactics) upon request.

At the conclusion of the season, candidates may email programs to remind them of their interest. Some programs also reach out to applicants via email or phone to offer them an opportunity to ask any last questions. Applicants are very sensitive to any perception of pressure to reveal their Match preferences, and program directors must remember that they are forbidden from asking applicants about these preferences or indicating an applicant's position on the program's list.

## The Rank Order List

Creation of the program's rank order list (ROL) can be a difficult process. Return to your program mission and what makes a resident most likely to succeed in your program. Program directors typically are unable to know how deep they will go into their list to fill their program each year. The NRMP uses a computerized matching algorithm that attempts to pair each applicant with their choices, in order, until the applicant is matched or all choices exhausted (National Resident Matching Program 2020). Initially, applicants are tentatively matched by the algorithm with the first program choice that has also ranked them, but they may be displaced by other applicants who rank higher on that program's ROL as slots become filled. The algorithm then attempts to pair any displaced applicants with their next-ranked programs. Thus, both programs and applicants benefit from ranking their true preferences in order on the ROL. An important consideration is who and how many people should view the final Match list. Remember that there is a potential impact if the applicant (who is also your future resident), a faculty member, or any co-residents learn an applicant's position on the list. Most programs therefore keep the final ROL and deliberations about admissions highly confidential. There are also regulations regarding creating the list in the system specified by the NRMP. Finally, be sure to certify your list in NRMP by the date specified; if your list is not certified, your program will not be included in the Match.

## Match Week

The NRMP publishes the Match Week schedule far in advance. Programs usually learn if they have been filled on Monday at 11 A.M. Eastern Standard Time. Unfilled programs and applicants then enter the Supplemental Offer and Acceptance Program (SOAP). Describing the full SOAP process is outside the scope of this chapter but should be reviewed in case your program does not fill or you are called upon to assist students who have not matched. On Thursday at 2 P.M. programs receive a confidential list of their matched applicants. Friday is "Match Day." At 12 P.M. students learn the name of the program to which they matched. At 1 P.M. applicant Match results are available in the "Registration, Ranking, and Results" (R3) software system and program Match results by ranked applicant reports are available.

Be sure to reach out to welcome your new residents! Plan to introduce them to each other, to the department, and to current residents by email. Send a thank you to everyone involved in the interview process to thank them for the conclusion of another Match cycle.

## Special Considerations

### *COUPLES MATCHING*

Applicants who choose to apply as a couple rank pairs of programs, instead of individual programs, with their partner. Ranking applicants higher or lower because they are part of a couple confers no advantage to programs. If both applicants are applying to your program, consider the potential conflicts of having a matched couple and discuss such concerns with your designated institutional officer prior to ranking.

### *TRANSFERS*

Each year, a number of residents desire to transfer between programs or specialties. Transfers may apply in the Match, but generally the process of interviewing and offering spots occurs outside of the Match process. The timing of acceptance may also occur independent of the usual July 1 start date. Programs should consult with their designated institutional officer and state licensing board and review the Accreditation Council for Graduate Medical Education (ACGME) program requirements when considering credit provided for prior training and to determine any applicable institutional and NRMP policies regarding transfer residents.

### *CLOSING HOSPITALS*

In the unfortunate event of a hospital closure, residents funded through the Center for Medicare Services at that hospital become "displaced" or "orphaned." Programs may either offer unfilled positions to orphaned applicants or apply to the ACGME for a temporary increase in spots in order to offer positions. The Center for Medicare Services–allotted monies for each resident slot accompanies orphaned residents to their new program for the duration of the resident's training. Because of the many factors involved and instability inherent to a closing hospital, programs accepting such residents will need to be in frequent communication with the designated institutional officer.

# STUDENT ADVISING

## Exploring Psychiatry as a Career

Medical students considering psychiatry often seek to gain more exposure to the field to see if it is the right specialty choice. Those applying to psychiatry may also ask for tips about how to be more competitive for residency. The number of students who enter medical school committed to psychiatry as a specialty is relatively low compared with the number who eventually choose psychiatry (Goldenberg et al. 2017), but approximately half of the students planning to pursue psychiatry at the start of medical school go on to psychiatry residencies. Your guidance can help students with this extremely important decision.

For students with an early interest in psychiatry who are not yet committed, learning about the specialty and how it compares with others may be helpful. The AAMC offers a "Careers in Medicine" program (www.aamc.org/cim) that offers a wealth of information about various specialties and subspecialties, as well as an assessment of students' interests, values, personality, and skills, that may help students identify a career path that fits these attributes. Additional ways to explore psychiatry as a career include the following.

### *JOINING THE AMERICAN PSYCHIATRIC ASSOCIATION AND STUDENT INTEREST GROUPS*

One of the best initial steps for a student with an interest in psychiatry is to join the American Psychiatric Association (APA; www.psychiatry.org/residents-medical-students/medical-students) or a psychiatry student interest group, if available. The APA offers free memberships to medical students, including osteopathic and international students. Benefits of student membership include free online access to the *American Journal of Psychiatry* and *Psychiatric News*, discounts on APA Publishing books and journals, and free registration for the APA annual meeting and Mental Health Services (formerly the Institute on Psychiatric Services) conference. The medical student section of the APA website links to various online resources for medical students and to the Psychiatry Student Interest Group Network (PsychSIGN; www.psychsign.org). Founded and supported by APA, PsychSIGN is "a national network of medical students interested in psychiatry, from those with a rough interest in the brain and mind to those already in the residency application and match process." PsychSIGN comprises psychiatry interest groups at medical schools from across the country, and membership is free for medical students. It also offers a newsletter of student-related content and free regional conferences open to students.

Psychiatry specialty organizations, such as the American Academy of Child and Adolescent Psychiatry (www.aacap.org/AACAP/Medical_Students_and_Residents/Medical_Students/Home.aspx) and Academy of Consultation-Liaison Psychiatry (www.clpsychiatry.org/about-aclp/join-aclp) offer free membership to medical students and an array of materials to help them better understand the subspecialties. Becoming a member of the APA and PsychSIGN also indicates interest in psychiatry on a residency application. Some schools have students take leadership roles in their student interest groups, and PsychSIGN has regional representatives and other leadership roles that offer students a broader array of experiences and add credibility to their residency application.

### *EARLY CLINICAL EXPERIENCE*

Preclinical students are usually most interested in an experience to see what psychiatrists actually do. The availability of such experiences varies widely. In many medical schools, organized preclinical student experiences provide some exposure to specialty fields, but many students spend the majority of their first 2 years in classroom settings with little clinical experience beyond basic interviewing and physical examination. In such circumstances, students typically seek some type of "shadowing" experience, such as attending clinical rounds with an inpatient or consultation-liaison service where clinical students and psychiatry residents are part of a team or following a faculty psychiatrist during clinical duties. Sometimes students shadow psychiatry residents on call, giving them both the opportunity to see psychiatry "in the trenches" and to talk with residents in depth about their decision to pursue psychiatry and their experience in residency. Faculty should check with their dean's office for particular policies or procedures for such clinical experiences outside of the standard clerkship rotations.

### *RESEARCH AND QUALITY IMPROVEMENT PROJECTS*

Involvement in research or quality improvement projects may also allow students to gain more experience in psychiatry and to meet psychiatry residents and faculty. Although quality research experiences may be difficult to find, many schools offer summer research positions. Industrious students may also find relevant research experiences by contacting faculty at their institution to see if paid or unpaid positions are available. Some departments of psychiatry have active quality improvement programs that may offer opportunities for student participation that are more flexible and time limited than typical research. Students should be aware that although research experiences may have some benefit to confirm their specialty choice and may improve their application, their primary focus should be on required courses and clerkships. The medical school transcript, MSPE, clinical letters of recommendation, and USMLE scores are likely to have more impact on their application unless they are planning a research career.

### *ADVOCACY AND SERVICE EXPERIENCES*

Advocacy and service-related experiences may help students learn more not only about psychiatry but also about mental health systems of care, stigma against those with mental illness, and the importance of public policy and government relations. Such opportunities run the gamut from medical school–associated free clinics with a mental health focus, to fundraising for various organizations, to direct involvement with local politicians and programs to improve the lives of people with mental illness. Organizations such as the American Foundation for Suicide Prevention (https://afsp.org/take-action) and National Alliance on Mental Illness (www.nami.org) have opportunities for volunteers to help with fundraising and with prevention and screening interventions and even to provide extra training or grant opportunities to start local projects. Leadership roles in advocacy or service organizations can point not only to applicants' depth of involvement but also to their substantial potential.

### *SOCIAL INTERACTIONS TO FIND THE BEST FIT*

One often underestimated impact on specialty choice is whether the students connect interpersonally with others in that profession. Each specialty in medicine has, to some degree, its own personality. Spending extra time with people who work in a given specialty may help students determine their best fit. Many departments of psychiatry offer opportunities in addition to the student interest group for students to interact with residents and faculty. Some proactive departments keep a list of interested students and invite them to departmental social gatherings and parties.

### *CONFIRMING INTEREST AND BUILDING AN APPLICATION*

Most medical students who pursue a residency in psychiatry make the decision during medical school; many point to the clerkship experience as the confirming or initiating event that solidified their interest. Often, this means that students determine psychiatry as a specialty choice late in the junior year. Once decided on psychiatry, students generally contact faculty with whom they rotated or that they had as teachers in earlier psychiatry-related courses for advice about how to improve their application for residency. Departments may designate specialty advisors, often clerkship directors, to assist in this process.

### *ELECTIVES AND ADDITIONAL EXPERIENCES*

For those who have narrowed their preferred specialty choices but have not yet committed, additional clinical experiences via electives or other opportunities may provide clarity. Electives in the senior year must be scheduled early, preferably before September, to allow students to confirm their specialty preference before residency applications are due. When a student's schedule does not allow this, creativity may be needed to identify additional clinical exposure outside of the standard curriculum. If available, students might take call with residents or round with attending physicians on weekends. Attending psychiatry interest group meetings, grand rounds, conferences, and department of psychiatry social gatherings may also be helpful.

Early electives are also important for students who have a confirmed interest in psychiatry. Letters of recommendation often come from supervising faculty on these rotations. Specialty rotations in psychiatry confirm a commitment to psychiatry on residency applications and provide more direct clinical experience that students can use on personal statements and during interviews.

## Advising for the Recruitment Process

Faculty advisors simultaneously serve as students' coach, mentor, and cheerleader during the interview and Match process. Following are the steps one should undertake when advising a student for the Match.

### *FAMILIARIZE YOURSELF WITH TIMELINES, RULES, AND REGULATIONS*

The NRMP publishes a timeline for the Match process yearly, but the true timeline for preparing applications begins around May of the year before a student applies. The NRMP updates its rules and list of prohibited actions at least annually.

### *FAMILIARIZE YOURSELF WITH RESOURCES*

For the past several years, the number of U.S. medical school graduates applying to a psychiatry residency has increased (American Psychiatric Association 2019). In addition to your counsel, students will be looking for resources to help guide them through the process. You should be aware of the sources of students' information. Medical students typically use several resources to aid in their application process. "A Roadmap to Psychiatry Residency" (www.psychiatry.org/residents-medical-students/medical-students/apply-for-psychiatric-residency) represents the work of a joint group of educators from numerous academic psychiatric organizations and national groups and provides a comprehensive overview for medical students of the timeline for the Match and guidance on topics such as writing letters of recommendation, personal statements, and what questions to ask on the interview day.

The AAMC offers two resources to help students applying for residency: Residency Explorer (www.residencyexplorer.org) and Apply Smart (https://students-residents.aamc.org/applying-residency/apply-smart-residency). Both contain data about previous years' Match outcomes that students can compare with their own data. Residency Explorer is in early testing at this time, and the AAMC is gathering feedback from students and program directors to improve the product. Other resources advertise that they help students make decisions about where to apply. Some use proprietary data and membership self-report, whereas others may contain completely student-created content.

Joining academic psychiatry organizations such as the Association of Academic Psychiatrists, Association of Directors of Medical Student Educators in Psychiatry, or AADPRT will help keep you abreast of trends in the application process and the emergence of new resources for students to review. The latter two organizations have very active listservs that can provide a faculty advisor with great knowledge and direction.

### *WORK WITH OTHER FACULTY ADVISORS*

Consider naming a core group of psychiatry educators to serve as faculty advisors. This group can work collaboratively to support each other and to provide guidance to students. A faculty advising group can also serve as an opportunity for junior faculty to become involved in education and learn about how to coach and advise students.

### *ADVISE STUDENTS ON HOW AND WHERE TO APPLY*

The number of students applying to psychiatry residency increased between 2012 and 2020 (Association of American Medical Colleges 2020a). Many students feel pressure about deciding how many programs they should apply to. There is no correct number of applications for any one applicant. The AAMC's Apply Smart data provide some statistics on the diminishing rate of return on the number of applications. Anxiety often drives the urge to apply to a large number of programs.

Encourage your applicants to think about the size of the residency, fellowship options, clinical sites or unique rotation opportunities, location of the program, and diversity of residents and faculty. Encourage them to be honest with themselves about their preferences. Students should review numerous websites and come up with a preliminary list for you to review.

### *ADVISE STUDENTS ON LETTERS OF RECOMMENDATION*

Encourage students to ask for recommendations early and to focus on asking people who can give them a positive letter of recommendation. Encourage students to choose a letter writer who knows them via clinical or research interactions and not just someone who may have name recognition in the field. Consider holding a letter-writing workshop in the department. Letters are often key to distinguishing applicants from one another, and the skills to craft these letters are generally not well known. Typically, applicants need three or four letters, and some programs may require letters from a primary care specialty or department chair. Encourage students to review prospective programs' websites for the latest requirements.

### *ADVISE STUDENTS ON PERSONAL STATEMENTS*

You will serve as editor and guide in the personal statements process. A personal statement serves many functions at once: it may provide information about the applicant and why he or she is a good fit for a career in psychiatry, discuss how the applicant chose psychiatry and future goals, and, if necessary, explain any obstacles or challenges that arose during medical school. Faculty advisors should encourage students to produce early drafts and should be prepared to meet with the students as they edit their statements. Often, early drafts of personal statements will look more like personal statements submitted for medical school. Discourage students from listing what is already in their ERAS application or from dwelling on negative or challenging aspects of their application. They should speak to their difficulties, what they have learned about themselves through the process of change, and how they plan to use their experience to become better psychiatrists.

Students may ask whether they should disclose sensitive topics in their personal statements, such as their ethnicity, immigrant status, mental health conditions, or sexual orientation. This is an individual decision, and they should consider the pros and cons. If they feel comfortable sharing this information and discussing it with (potentially) every person with whom they interview, then they may share their experiences. On the other hand, if they are still processing these experiences and are not comfortable with that level of self-disclosure, that is acceptable as well. The choice to divulge sensitive information and how to divulge it in a residency application is personal, and advice regarding it should be similarly sensitive and individualized.

### *PREPARING STUDENTS FOR THE INTERVIEW DAY*

As mentioned, resources exist that provide students guidance on the nuts and bolts of the interview day. Remind your students about professionalism and that the interview begins with their first contacts with the program or any of the program's residents and concludes with the close of the interview day. Any interactions they have, even with people who are not residents or faculty, may impact where the program ranks them.

Some institutions and departments offer medical students an opportunity to do "mock" interviews. Faculty, senior residents, or residents interested in academic careers interview students to practice their answers and provide them with meaningful feedback. This must be done with some care if students are applying to your own program. If you choose as a department to offer mock interviews, make sure to separate members who are involved in the "mock" interview process from those who are involved in residency selection.

### *ADVISE ON POSTINTERVIEW COMMUNICATIONS*

Some students ask about contact with a program after the interview. This may be done as a thank you or as a way to let the program know of their interest. Psychiatry program directors differ on this topic; some programs outright discourage postinterview communications, whereas others have no preference. If the program's website offers clear guidance, encourage students to follow such guidance. Thank you notes are generally encouraged.

### *ADVISE STUDENTS WHO ARE AT RISK OF NOT MATCHING*

Some students will have academic "bumps and bruises" on their application, such as low scores, a leave of absence, or a failed clerkship. These students may need to apply to more programs or to programs that have not been very competitive historically. They will also need to speak to their challenges in their personal statement and be prepared to speak about them during interviews. During competitive Match years, applicants with particularly challenging applications should consider applying to backup specialties.

You may need to prepare your student to send letters to residency programs asking that their application be considered. Encourage them to write succinct emails speaking to their specific interest in that residency program. Some faculty advisors have also been sending personal letters to individuals in residency programs with whom they are acquainted in order to advocate for a review of their student. There have been various responses and successes in doing this, but given the avalanche of applications, such approaches may be important for students with challenging applications.

### *ADVISE STUDENTS IN THE SUPPLEMENTAL OFFER AND ACCEPTANCE PROGRAM*

The SOAP is a high-stress environment. Students must move quickly from shock and mourning about not matching to recovery and change. Work closely with your dean of student affairs and try to make yourself available in person or by phone for the duration of Match week. Work with your advisees to take stock of what is available in the SOAP. In recent Match cycles, preliminary and transitional-year positions have been more abundant than categorical positions in SOAP. Work with your advisee to develop a short- and long-term plan for securing a medical career. Once SOAP is completed—regardless of outcome—you may want to meet with your advisee to discuss their challenges in the application process. This gives the advisee a chance to reflect on any missteps and to develop a plan. This also provides you, as the advisor, information to better inform the next round of applicants.

### Addressing Dual Relationships

What if you serve as the faculty advisor and are also your institution's psychiatry residency program director? How do you navigate this dual relationship? This situation requires full disclosure by the program director and a clear understanding of expectations. Program directors who serve as faculty advisors must make it clear to their trainees that these are separate roles and that advising does not guarantee the trainees' acceptance to the home program. Alternatively, whenever possible, program directors can choose to avoid faculty advising and instead set up an advising group of other psychiatry educators. This may shield them from concerns of bias.

## CONCLUSION

Both recruitment and student advising are important, exciting, and challenging roles. Both require that faculty stay current with national trends and NRMP rules and are best achieved through collaborative departmental efforts and advance planning.

## — KEY POINTS —

- Successful residency recruitment is time intensive and requires attention to departmental mission and advanced planning.
- Serving as a faculty advisor is a multifaceted role. Familiarize yourself with the rules of the Match process and be mindful of dual relationships if you will serve as both program director and faculty advisor.
- Students interested in psychiatry should consider free membership in the American Psychiatric Association or one of several psychiatry subspecialty organizations that offer access to journals and various student-specific information.
- Advocacy, quality improvement, and research experiences related to mental health can be a great way for students to learn more about psychiatry while also adding interest to their application.

## REFERENCES

Aibana O, Swails J, Flores R, Love L: Bridging the gap: holistic review to increase diversity in graduate medical education. Acad Med 94(8):1137–1141, 2019

American Psychiatric Association: 2018 Resident-Fellow Census. American Psychiatric Association, Washington, DC, 2019. Available at: https://www.psychiatry.org/File%20Library/Residents-MedicalStudents/Residents/APA-Resident-Census-2019.pdf. Accessed September 30, 2019.

Association of American Medical Colleges: ERAS Statistics (website). Association of American Medical Colleges, 2020a. Available at: https://www.aamc.org/data-reports/interactive-data/eras-statistics-data. Accessed November 30, 2020.

Association of American Medical Colleges: Holistic Review (website). Association of American Medical Colleges, 2020b. Available at: https://www.aamc.org/services/member-capacity-building/holistic-review. Accessed February 14, 2020.

Boyse TD, Patterson SK, Cohan RH, et al: Does medical school performance predict radiology resident performance? Acad Radiol 9(4):437–445, 2002

Brenner AM, Mathai S, Jain S, Mohl PC: Can we predict "problem residents"? Acad Med 85(7):1147–1151, 2010

Goldenberg MN, Williams DK, Spollen JJ: Stability of and factors related to medical student specialty choice of psychiatry. Am J Psychiatry 174(9):859–866, 2017

Hartman ND, Lefebvre CW, Manthey DE: A narrative review of the evidence supporting factors used by residency program directors to select applicants for interviews. J Grad Med Educ 11(3):268–273, 2019

National Resident Matching Program: Results and Data: 2019 Main Residency Match. Washington, DC, National Resident Matching Program, 2019

National Resident Matching Program: How the Matching Algorithm Works. NRMP website, 2020. Available at: http://www.nrmp.org/matching-algorithm. Accessed February 14, 2020.

Papadakis MA, Teherani A, Banach MA, et al: Disciplinary action by medical boards and prior behavior in medical school. N Engl J Med 353(25):2673–2682, 2005

Raman T, Alrabaa RG, Sood A, et al: Does residency selection criteria predict performance in orthopaedic surgery residency? Clin Orthop Relat Res 474:908–914, 2016

Stohl HE, Hueppchen NA, Bienstock JL: Can medical school performance predict residency performance? Resident selection and predictors of successful performance in obstetrics and gynecology. J Grad Med Educ 2(3):322–326, 2010

Taylor TE, Milem JF, Coleman AL: Bridging the Research to Practice Gap: Achieving Mission-Driven Diversity and Inclusion Goals. A Review of Research Findings and Policy Implications for Colleges and Universities. New York, The College Board, 2016

Zuckerman SL, Kelly PD, Dewan MC, et al: Predicting resident performance from preresidency factors: a systematic review and applicability to neurosurgical training. World Neurosurg 110:475–484, 2018

# CHAPTER 10

# EVALUATION STRATEGIES

Alex Loeks-Johnson, M.D.
Lora Wichser, M.D.

## ASSESSMENT AND EVALUATION STRATEGIES

When designing a psychiatric course or clerkship, it is important to be aware of the difference between "assessment" and "evaluation." *Assessment*, or *formative assessment*, is the observation and study of students' learning and performance with the primary goal of enhancing student education. *Evaluation*, or "summative assessment," describes the final determination of student performance that dictates both the grade and whether the student's performance is high enough to pass the course and move on to more challenging material (Morgenstern 2019). Because most clinical clerkships assess and evaluate a broader set of skills than classroom-based courses, this chapter primarily focuses on assessment and evaluation tools for clinical clerkships. However, much of the content in this chapter applies to classroom-based courses as well.

### Assessment

Because the goal of student assessment is to enhance education and performance, many accrediting and administrative bodies recognize it as an essential tool in medical student education. For example, the Liaison Committee on Medical Education (LCME) requires mandatory formative assessment in clinical clerkships in the form of midrotation feedback, with a primary goal of identifying students who are struggling

(Konopasek et al. 2016; Morgenstern 2019). The primary goals of identifying struggling students are to reduce course failures and poor grades and to protect patient safety, but it does not help guide further education of the average or above-average students who are not struggling. As such, it is important to recognize the need for other systems of assessment to help all students maximize their performance.

Unfortunately, methods of assessment are often used simply as a snapshot of students' performance and not used to meaningfully alter their educational plan (Konopasek et al. 2016). Ideally, all data from formative assessments would produce valuable feedback to guide future education and create a cycle of improvement and reassessment. This assessment model, although more informative than many in use today, requires a significant time and energy investment from administration, faculty, and students.

Assessment of students during the psychiatry clerkship primarily comes in the form of observation and feedback regarding clinical skills, knowledge, and attitudes, such as in their patient interviews and treatment plans. This style of assessment has high feasibility and practicality and can offer large amounts of actionable feedback for improvement. Such assessment is generally informal, with rapid feedback after each encounter, but more structured methods are also available. If the clerkship contains a final evaluation of medical knowledge (e.g., a multiple-choice examination) more focused methods to assess knowledge may be in place, such as computerized pretests or assignments, and should be used to guide curriculum.

Structured methods are available for assessing the clinical skills used in clerkships. Three well-known examples are the Objective Structured Clinical Examinations (OSCEs), the mini-Clinical Evaluation Exercise (mini-CEX), and entrustable professional activities (EPAs). OSCEs are a set of clinical interviews, physical examinations, and treatment plans that occur with standardized patients, actors trained to portray a certain medical illness or condition (Morgenstern 2019). Because students are assessed on interviews, examination skills, and treatment planning, OSCEs have the advantage of simultaneously assessing both clinical skills and medical knowledge. The standardized patients are instructed to give the same presentation to all students to make the assessment of relative performance more valid. However, OSCEs are resource and time intensive, students can feel that interviews with standardized patients do not reflect how they relate to real patients, and grading performance and giving feedback take a significant amount of time.

The mini-CEX is a real clinical encounter that is monitored and evaluated by preceptors. Although predominantly a tool to evaluate resident physicians, it has recently been used in the assessment of medical students as well (Morgenstern 2019). A relative advantage of the mini-CEX is that it involves real patients instead of trained actors, which avoids the lack of realism found in OSCEs. Due to its brevity (one patient encounter with one student), feedback can occur immediately afterward, allowing the student to build on this feedback throughout the rotation.

EPAs are a new strategy for capturing clinical assessments developed to support competency-based medical education. EPAs are a system for quantifying how much the preceptor trusts the learner to perform a given task (Ten Cate et al. 2016). Preceptors use a scale of trustworthiness, which translates into level of supervision required to complete the task, to assign a perceived level of proficiency in certain tasks (Englander et al. 2016). Some medical schools are moving toward capturing EPAs as a method of ensuring that all graduates are ready for residency.

## Evaluation

Evaluation, or summative assessment, most commonly occurs at the end of the course and generally consists of data from multiple components, such as written examinations, written submissions (e.g., case report, reflection essay, research topics), and subjective evaluations by the preceptors. In essence, the overall goal of student *assessment* is to enhance students' learning and skills to maximize their performance on the end-of-course *evaluations*.

An end-of-rotation evaluation system should evaluate all necessary components of student performance and maximize chances of success by incorporating information learned from prior assessment tools. As such, final evaluations are often most valid when several sources evaluating different areas of competency are utilized and combined. We review the two most common methods of student assessment: multiple choice tests and preceptor feedback.

### *MULTIPLE-CHOICE TESTS*

Generally, the format and content of final examinations are at the discretion of the clerkship director, although the governing medical school may have policies surrounding end-of-rotation examinations. The most common method is multiple-choice testing. Essay examinations obtain a more accurate representation of a student's knowledge but are time consuming to grade and more prone to subjective evaluation. Multiple-choice tests are far easier to score, and results are more generalizable and objective between students. Interestingly, students enrolled in higher education tend to prefer multiple-choice tests over essays (Struyven et al. 2005) because they are thought to be more forgiving.

Clerkship directors may choose between preexisting, standardized national tests, such as the National Board of Medical Examiners (NBME) subject examinations, or local preceptor-generated tests. NBME subject examinations are computerized multiple-choice tests designed to evaluate students' medical knowledge and clinical decision making. Questions are generally vignette style, and the overall format is very similar to the U.S. Medical Licensing Examination (USMLE) Step examinations. Reliability and validity of the NBME examination are high. If purchased, the NBME also provides score guidelines that detail past performance of students, trends, and suggestions for pass, failure, and honors designations (Morgenstern 2019). However, the NBME tests are quite expensive, have rigid administration requirements, and may not evaluate the exact topics the course director values. Thus, many course directors create their own or use a nationally produced, discipline-specific examination. Benefits to this method include reduced cost and the ability to tailor content to specific material. However, examinations created by a preceptor tend to have lower reliability and reproducibility and may suffer from poorly written questions if preceptors are not trained in creating multiple-choice questions (Morgenstern 2019).

### *PRECEPTOR FEEDBACK*

As mentioned, feedback from the observing preceptors is often used as both a tool for student assessment and a portion of the student's final evaluation. As such, it is essential that all preceptors who observe, assess, and evaluate students be trained in the expectations for each student. For example, preceptors should have knowledge of the preclinical course content so as not to judge students too harshly or teach below the student's knowledge level. Preceptors should have different expectations for different levels of students (e.g., third-year students on core clerkship, students on electives, students on a subinternship). It is essential that clerkship directors monitor evaluation trends among different preceptors to ensure fairness and validity in student grading by determining whether certain preceptors tend to grade more or less harshly than others. The more formalized the feedback system is among preceptors, the more objective and valid the feedback will be. An example of a formalized feedback system would be the EPAs mentioned earlier, which are often used as both assessment and evaluation tools.

Finally, clerkship evaluations should be accompanied by a narrative assessment consisting of statements from preceptors who worked with the student. This can further accentuate the students' strengths and delineate areas for improvement. Certain portions of the narrative assessment, often strengths and areas of high performance, may be included in the Medical Student Performance Evaluation letter, which is essential for residency applications. Other portions of the narrative assessment may be confidential and shared only with the student and clerkship director.

# PRACTICAL CONSIDERATIONS FOR ASSESSMENT AND EVALUATION

## The Final Grade

The goal of these methods of evaluation is to produce a quantifiable measure of students' performance, assign grades, and determine whether the students have passed or failed. The style of grading varies widely among clerkships. For example, a 2012 study of clerkship grading practices of U.S. medical schools found massive heterogeneity among grading schemes between different schools and even among clerkships at the same school (Alexander et al. 2012). In the 119 medical schools evaluated, eight grading systems were discovered. The most common was a 4-tier system (e.g., A/B/C/F, honors/high pass/pass/fail), but they ranged from 2-tier (pass/fail) to 11-tier. The percentage of students receiving the highest grade in the clerkship ranged from 2% to 93%, and the vast majority of students received a grade in the top three tiers no matter how many total tiers were present.

One can imagine the confusion of residency admission committees trying to discover the meaning of a clerkship grade when comparing applicants from different schools. Important considerations when designing a grading style include the number of grading tiers, whether students' performances will be curved (e.g., a set percentage of students in each tier) or evaluated on absolute scores, and developing clear, coherent language to define the tiers (Morgenstern 2019). Often, the medical school itself will have guidelines for grading schemes of core rotations, but elective courses may have more flexibility.

## Diversity in the Clinical Environment

Students who come from a minority background require intentional assessments, particularly in clinical settings that may be inherently unwelcoming to underrepresented minority students. Because psychiatry depends so heavily on interpersonal communication skills, subjective evaluations of students will likely focus on this aspect of patient and team-based care. Students who feel they are discriminated against or feel less accepted in clinical settings, such as ethnic or LGBTQI minorities, or who have their own lived experience with psychiatric illness may have difficulty fully expressing themselves and interacting with patients and team members. At this point, it will be unclear if they truly lack interpersonal skills or if their environment is preventing them from showcasing their skills. Either way, it will be difficult for these students to perform adequately, and their clerkship evaluations will likely suffer.

The primary method to alleviate this issue is to conscientiously create an environment that allows all students to feel safe and supported. Preceptors must address upsetting incidents that may occur, such as racially or sexually inappropriate comments by a patient. Explicitly state that student discomfort with a patient will not be regarded negatively. Students commonly describe unreported and unaddressed discrimination toward medical students on clerkships (Hardeman et al. 2016). Medical students must understand that anonymous and effective measures are available that can be undertaken to correct such behavior, with *no* risk for retaliation. Most medical schools have preexisting programs to protect students from discrimination, and clerkship administrators should emphasize and augment these programs.

## Components of Successful Assessments

The 2010 Ottawa Conference on the Assessment of Competence in Medicine and the Healthcare Professions released key components of a good assessment methodology (Norcini et al. 2011). Clerkship administrators should ensure these criteria are met when designing and implementing assessment strategies.

1. **Validity and coherence:** The assessment modality must be evidence based to provide valid results that can be used to enhance learning.
2. **Reproducibility and consistency:** The same results should be expected if the assessment were repeated under similar circumstances.
3. **Equivalence:** The assessment should produce similar results at different sites and cycles.
4. **Feasibility:** Performing the assessment should be reasonable and practical. In clinical settings, everyone is busy; therefore, a shorter assessment is more feasible.
5. **Educational effect:** Students should be motivated to prepare for the assessment in a way that enhances their education and has lasting benefit.
6. **Catalytic effect:** The results of the assessment should identify areas of strength and weakness to motivate and guide future learning.
7. **Acceptability:** All stakeholders in the assessment process (e.g., preceptors, students, patients) should feel that the assessment is credible and useful.

### Dangers of the Likert Scale

Clinical assessment (and often evaluation) tools commonly use Likert-type scales, rating items on a scale of one to four, with each number corresponding to a response, such as "does not meet expectations," "meets expectations," "above expectations," "far exceeds expectations," and so on. Many evaluators circle all high numbers, due to the (often correct) perception that an evaluation could "make or break" students' access to matching into the specialty of their choice. Many specialties require a top-tier grade (e.g., honors) for an applicant to qualify for a residency interview. The danger of a Likert scale is that when a student's future is on the line, it will bias the preceptor toward higher ratings. The end result is that intraclerkship performance will often be overestimated, and students may feel justifiably upset that their final evaluation scores can be significantly lower than predicted based on prior assessments. Many medical schools are moving toward a pass/not yet system for this reason, among many.

## IDENTIFICATION AND ASSISTANCE OF THE STRUGGLING LEARNER

Arguably, the most important function of formative assessments is to identify struggling students. The stakes for poor performance on a clinical rotation are high, ranging from a poor grade, to needing to repeat the clerkship and delaying graduation, to expulsion from the medical school if this is a continued pattern. Here we review the basic steps involved in identifying and assisting struggling students.

### Identification

Many clerkships have adopted a competency-based assessment system with components that are similar to the Accreditation Council for Graduate Medical Education's core competencies used to evaluate resident physicians, such as "medical knowledge," "interpersonal and communication skills," and "professionalism" (Swick et al. 2006). A struggling learner may have deficiencies in one or more competency domains, and faculty and staff working with the student must identify these deficiencies as soon as possible. As described earlier, the LCME has mandated that all clerkship students receive midrotation feedback (Konopasek et al. 2016), but midrotation can be too late to create a comprehensive improvement plan. Two factors are critical to increasing the chances of early identification. First, all faculty, staff, and residents working with students should receive training on how to identify struggling learners and notify appropriate clerkship leadership. Second, reliable, valid, and robust assessment tools should be used with the goal of distinguishing students who will likely struggle if no intervention is implemented.

When choosing formative assessment tools, a primary goal is to be able to identify struggling learners as early as possible to maximize chances of intraclerkship improvement and avoid failures and repeats. Exactly when a struggling student comes to the attention of clerkship administrators is highly variable. Medical schools vary as to whether they have programs in place to alert clerkship administration of incoming students who have struggled previously so that the school can help them prepare educational resources for this student. Although such programs have advantages, many schools have barred the practice out of fear that they could create a negative bias about a student before the next clerkship. Some clerkships encourage students who have struggled in the past to speak privately and preemptively with clerkship administration to create an education plan.

## Investigation

Once a student is identified as struggling, it is essential to thoroughly clarify the nature, causes, and perceptions of the problem, using information from both the student and those observing the student, as well as historical and environmental data, if applicable. Clinical clerkships present new challenges that were not present in the preclinical years of medical school. Clerkships require that students integrate themselves and work well in a medical team. Their interpersonal interactions with patients and other medical professionals are rigorously evaluated in ways not possible in preclinical years. In addition, simply working in a hospital for the first time is a difficult transition. A 2017 survey of medical students on their first hospital-based clerkships revealed that most students struggle with navigating a large, new hospital, identifying and physically locating patients, and adapting to the new style of teaching and learning that clinical medicine offers (Barrett et al. 2017).

Especially important for clerkship administrators is to assess how the assessment and evaluation of students differ across faculty, residents, and clinical sites. For example, a 2015 paper examining medical students on their emergency medicine rotation revealed that increased emergency department overcrowding (e.g., higher patient volume, reduced physical space, and less time with attending physicians) was associated with decreased student performance on end-of-rotation examinations and with poorer student evaluations of the rotation (Wei et al. 2015). This paper suggests it is critical to properly titrate student workload and develop a physical learning environment that emphasizes learning and performance. In addition, evaluations differ between raters, and clerkship administrators must attempt to standardize student assessments and evaluation as much as possible.

Finally, the psychiatry rotation itself can present many new challenges and obstacles to students. Students are often pushed out of their comfort zones because psychiatric patients, whether agitated, psychotic, manic, or cognitively impaired, can be quite difficult to interview. Interviews often touch on subjects that are taboo in our society, such as suicide, sex, substance use, and violence. It is easy to see how students who perform exceptionally well in other clerkships could struggle in psychiatry, given the drastically different patient population and style of data gathering. Prepare students by offering information on mental status examination and interview skills and by modeling interviews with difficult patients.

Clerkship administration must review multiple sources of evidence, including objective data (e.g., graded assignments, OSCEs, structured interviews, final examination scores), comments from faculty and resident evaluators, and, arguably most important, the students themselves. Although outside the scope of this chapter, several examples of structured student interviews are available to assess students' insight of their struggles and the causes (Morgenstern 2019). Because the stakes of poor clerkship performance are so high, developing an in-depth portrait of a struggling student's strengths and weaknesses is essential, more so than for average students. Accurately detail exactly which areas must be addressed (e.g., medical knowledge, professionalism) in order to guide improvement efforts.

## Creation of Improvement Plan

The next step is for all involved parties, including clerkship administration, faculty and residents working with the student, and the student him- or herself, is to collaborate on the development of an improvement plan. Individual medical schools may have additional requirements, such as involvement from the student's faculty advisor or the dean for student affairs. Ideally, these steps will be taken early enough in the rotation to allow intrarotation improvement and to prevent examination or clerkship failure.

An individualized learning plan should then be created that is tailored to the individual student and the areas he or she is struggling in

(Morgenstern 2019). Such learning plans detail the goals, expectations, and plan for successful improvement. Document details of the specific areas of deficit, along with concrete and practical goals to bring the student's performance up to an acceptable level. The specific assessment strategies used to measure the student's performance and improvement and the learning strategies to be utilized should be described. Finally, the particulars of required, regular feedback sessions should be addressed, such as frequency and who will be present. Collaboration with the student is essential to maximize opportunities for self-assessment and self-directed learning, which allows the student to develop strategies to help identify and address future struggles, as well as the current problems.

## Implementation and Reassessment

Those involved in assessing and evaluating the student must be made aware of these goals—while maximizing the student's privacy as much as possible—to help the student reach them. It is most useful to identify one person, whether the clerkship director or a primary faculty evaluator, to have scheduled feedback sessions to review progress in the individualized learning plan. Changes to the plan can be made after rounds of feedback, assessment, and (hopefully) improvement. Ideally, feedback sessions will contain a review of objective and qualitative data from assessments, as well as a self-assessment by the student to identify progress made and areas that still need improvement, and the development of concrete goals that can be achieved by the next session. These feedback sessions should encourage a cycle of self-assessment, development of a plan to improve in problem areas, and implementation of the plan, followed by another round of self-assessment. This cycle should continue until all goals of the learning plan have been met and the relevant evaluators (e.g., student, faculty, residents, and clerkship director) agree that the student's performance is now satisfactory.

The assessment tools available in this phase are generally the same as those described earlier. However, during an improvement process they should be performed more frequently, accompanied by more feedback, and tailored to the specific problems with which the student is struggling. The student should not feel that he or she is being constantly tested. Instead, assessment tools should identify both strengths and weakness, and the student should be given both supportive and constructive feedback. During this process, it is preferable to use assessment tools that use direct observation and immediate feedback. For example, if a student is struggling with medical knowledge, an oral examination and case-based discussion should be chosen over a computerized multiple choice (Morgenstern 2019).

### Failing Grades

Unfortunately, course directors must prepare for the inevitability that a small number of students will receive grades or evaluations that necessitate a "failing" grade. This outcome can be devastating for the student, resulting in possible disciplinary action, course repeats, reduced performance in the residency Match, or expulsion. As mentioned, the reasons for course failure may be a combination of student factors (e.g., issues with medical knowledge, motivation, professionalism) and course factors (i.e., insufficient assessment and remediation tools). The next steps in this situation are varied and likely will also be influenced by medical school policy.

Failing grades likely require notification and further guidance from medical school administration, such as offices for student affairs or student advisors. A detailed review of student performance in the course is generally required, with input from the student and evaluators and objective data such as test results. The specific type of course will also dictate future remediation efforts. For example, a failing grade in a preclinical, lecture-based course may be remediated by retaking the final examination after a period of course review. More severe deficits may necessitate repeating the course the next time it is offered. Required core-clerkships likely have a more detailed policy for course failures than do elective clerkships, as dictated by medical school policy. If it is deemed necessary for a student to repeat a clinical clerkship, the more robust and frequent regimen of assessment, feedback, and reassessment designed for struggling students (as detailed earlier) should be implemented as soon as the student restarts the clerkship.

## CONCLUSION

When creating a psychiatry course for medical students, it is essential to implement systems for assessment and evaluation that are appropriate to the content students will be taught and that maximize the chances for student learning and success. *Assessment* refers to the process of determining students' knowledge, performance, and progress during the course, with the main goals of maximizing learning and increasing performance on end-of-course examinations or evaluations. The best assessment tools are practical and produce actionable feedback as to areas of student excellence and struggle. Assessment tools should ideally be used sufficiently to create a cycle of feedback and improvement and to identify struggling students sufficiently early to allow for performance improvement. *Evaluation* most commonly refers to end-of-rotation examinations or evaluations that generally dictate the final grade. Final evaluations should build on the material and concepts assessed throughout the clerkship, and the format of the final evaluation should be similar to that of prior assessment tools. Course directors, in conjunction with medical school input, should also develop a system for remediation for struggling students that includes more frequent and robust cycles of assessment and feedback.

## — KEY POINTS —

- Medical school psychiatry courses should have systems for student assessment and evaluation that measure course knowledge, progress, and performance.
- *Assessment* refers to the study of student knowledge and performance during a course, with the main goals of identifying areas for future teaching and detecting struggling students.
- *Evaluation* most often refers to end-of-course examinations or evaluations that determine students' final grade in the course.
- Assessment tools should be used to maximize performance on end-of-rotation evaluations and to identify struggling students early enough to allow for remediation to avoid course failures.

# REFERENCES

Alexander EK, Osman NY, Walling JL, Mitchell VG: Variation and imprecision of clerkship grading in U.S. medical schools. Acad Med 87(8):1070–1076, 2012

Barrett J, Trumble SC, McColl G: Novice students navigating the clinical environment in an early medical clerkship. Med Educ 51:1014–1024, 2017

Englander R, Flynn T, Call S, et al: Toward defining the foundation of the MD degree: core entrustable professional activities for entering residency. Acad Med 91(10):1352–1358, 2016

Hardeman RR, Przedworski JM, Burke S, et al: Association between perceived medical school diversity climate and change in depressive symptoms among medical students: a report from the Medical Student CHANGE Study. J Natl Med Assoc 108(4):225–235, 2016

Konopasek L, Norcini J, Krupat E: Focusing on the formative: building an assessment system aimed at student growth and development. Acad Med 91(11):1492–1497, 2016

Morgenstern BZ: Guidebook for Clerkship Directors, 5th Edition. North Syracuse, NY, Alliance for Clinical Education, 2019

Norcini J, Anderson B, Bollela V, Burch V, et al: Criteria for good assessment: consensus statement and recommendations from the Ottawa 2010 conference. Med Teach 33(3):206–214, 2011

Struyven K, Dochy F, Janssens S: Students' perceptions about evaluation and assessment in higher education: a review. Assessment and Evaluation in Higher Education 30(4):325–341, 2005

Swick S, Hall S, Beresin E: Assessing the ACGME competencies in psychiatry training programs. Acad Psychiatry 30(4):330–351, 2006

Ten Cate O, Hart D, Ankel F, et al: Entrustment decision making in clinical training. Acad Med 91(2):191–198, 2016

Wei G, Arya R, Ritz ZT, et al: How does emergency department crowding affect medical student test scores and clerkship evaluations? West J Emerg Med 16(6):913–918, 2015

# PART III

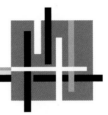

# RESIDENT AND FELLOWSHIP EDUCATION

## CHAPTER 11

# CURRICULUM

## Begin With the End

Jacqueline A. Hobbs, M.D., Ph.D.
Robert N. Averbuch, M.D.
Richard C. Holbert, M.D.
Gary L. Kanter, M.D.
Herbert E. Ward Jr., M.D.

**One** of the most challenging of the many jobs of a residency training director, whether new or experienced, is to develop the curriculum. For those who are new to the job, even defining what curriculum is may be difficult. Change is hard, and even experienced program directors may find revising or updating curriculum burdensome.

Our program is a medium to large program at the University of Florida in Gainesville, and we want to share our experiences with curriculum development and reform, both practical and conceptual. Our vision of curriculum development is as a long-term culture change, a big vision of where we want to be.

---

We would like to thank Mrs. Britany Ratliff, Mrs. Terry Lemesh, and Mrs. Dorothy McCallister, who provided clerical assistance with this chapter manuscript.

# WHAT IS CURRICULUM?

First, we want to have a consistent definition of *curriculum*. In clinical training, the term usually refers to both experiential and didactic learning. For adult learners, experiential is and should be the preponderance of the curriculum. Didactic learning should play a foundational role on which clinical learning is built and reinforced.

It is equally important to speak openly and frequently with faculty and residents about the dual nature of curriculum. Why? Faculty and residents often see curriculum as something you do in the classroom setting, droning on like the teacher in *Ferris Bueller's Day Off*, based on prior experiences in traditional medical education. Residents may look at the didactic time, often no more than 10%–20% of the week, and the limited number of topics covered and think that they are not learning enough. Residents commonly see clinical work as "service" and not as "education" or curriculum. Most clinical educators know that nothing could be further from the truth. Clinical rotations must have goals and objectives and reading assignments (book chapters and journal articles) to emphasize this point. Open discussion about the dual nature of curriculum can help both learner and teacher see that balancing these two components is essential.

# WHAT DOES THE ACGME SAY ABOUT CURRICULUM?

A well-known designated institutional official and former program director advised new program directors at our institution to read the Accreditation Council for Graduate Medical Education (ACGME) program requirements at the beginning of every academic year and anytime an update occurs and to reread them if they have a question. It is amazing how requirements can be forgotten or can seem clearer when read again or with a specific question in mind. The ACGME Psychiatry Program Requirements, Frequently Asked Questions, and Milestones (Table 11–1) are major resources for guiding curriculum development, especially for a new program director. Once the requirements are met, program directors and faculty are free to innovate.

There can be flexibility in what the curriculum emphasizes, according to the ACGME requirements. For example, if a program aims to produce physician-scientists, the curriculum would obviously be different from that of a program that aims to produce clinician-educators or community psychiatrists. Each would still have foundational knowledge that all psychiatrists need to know, but otherwise the program is free to

**Table 11–1.** Helpful resources for curriculum development

| Organization | Websites and pages[a] | Description/Notes |
|---|---|---|
| Accreditation Council for Graduate Medical Education | www.acgme.org | Main site[b]; provides general training information and resources (see "Program Directors and Coordinators" tab) |
| Clinical Learning Environment Review | www.acgme.org/What-We-Do/Initiatives/Clinical-Learning-Environment-Review-CLER | |
| Psychiatry | www.acgme.org/Specialties/Overview/pfcatid/21 | Psychiatry-specific information and requirements, frequently asked questions, and milestones |
| Self-Study | www.acgme.org/What-We-Do/Accreditation/Self-Study | Self-study information and tools |
| American Academy of Child and Adolescent Psychiatry | www.aacap.org | Main site[b]; Click "Member Resources" tab, then "Education Center" |
| American Association of Directors of Psychiatric Residency Training | www.aadprt.org | Click "Training Directors" tab |
| Curriculum Committee | www.aadprt.org/training-directors/curriculum | List of available peer-reviewed model curricula; tips on developing a curriculum |
| Important links | www.aadprt.org/training-directors/important-links | Links to other training organizations with curricular resources |
| Virtual Training Office | www.aadprt.org/training-directors/virtual-training-office | Repository of teaching/training materials |

**Table 11–1.** Helpful resources for curriculum development *(continued)*

| Organization | Websites and pages[a] | Description/Notes |
|---|---|---|
| American Board of Psychiatry and Neurology | www.abpn.com | Main site[b] |
| Taking a Specialty Exam > Psychiatry | www.abpn.com/become-certified/taking-a-specialty-exam/psychiatry | "Content Specifications" provides link to a PDF with all of content topics and their approximate weight on the certification examination[c] |
| American College of Psychiatrists | www.acpsych.org/prite | Psychiatry Resident-In-Training Examination (PRITE) |
| PRITE Content Outline | www.acpsych.org/content/documents/prite_content_outline_with_annotations_dec_2019.doc | |
| American Psychiatric Association | www.psychiatry.org | Main site[b] |
| Learning Center | www.psychiatry.org/psychiatrists/education/apa-learning-center | Provides learning modules/videos for residents and faculty development, continuing medical education, and self-assessment |
| Ethics | www.psychiatry.org/psychiatrists/practice/ethics | Ethics education materials |
| American Society of Clinical Psychopharmacology | https://ascpp.org/ | Main site[b] |
| Model Psychopharmacology Curriculum | https://ascpp.org/resources/educational-resource/ascp-model-psychopharmacology-curriculum-seventh-edition/ | Available for a fee; now in its tenth edition |

**Table 11–1.** Helpful resources for curriculum development *(continued)*

| Organization | Websites and pages[a] | Description/Notes |
|---|---|---|
| Association for Academic Psychiatry | www.academicpsychiatry.org | Main site[b] |
| Career Development | www.academicpsychiatry.org/career-development/ | Links to Master Educator program and other resources |
| Association of American Medical Colleges | www.aamc.org | Main site[b] |
| MedEdPortal | www.mededportal.org | Peer-reviewed, open-access teaching and assessment resources; more focus on undergraduate medical education |
| Medical Education | www.aamc.org/what-we-do/mission-areas/medical-education | |
| Association of Directors of Medical Student Education in Psychiatry | www.admsep.org | Main site[b] |
| Public Educational Resources | www.admsep.org/resources.php?c=public-resources | Includes self-directed and other learning modules; focus is on medical student education, but overlaps with residency education |
| National Neuroscience Curriculum Initiative | www.nncionline.org | Neuroscience curriculum and learning modules for residency training |

[a]Accessed November 27, 2020.
[b]Also linked from the American Association of Directors of Psychiatric Residency Training website.
[c]Examination content may change from time to time, so it is prudent to review regularly for updates.

innovate. The six ACGME core competencies must be incorporated into all program curricula and are especially emphasized in developing the goals and objectives (discussed further in Chapter 5). The curriculum must be organized, provide certain clinical experiences, and be assessed at least annually, usually during the ACGME required annual program evaluation.

Now that you know all the curriculum requirements, what are you waiting for? You've got this, right? Well, it is not easy. In fact, it can seem quite daunting. Other layers to good curriculum development exist that are not really spelled out in a list of requirements. We thought we would tell the story of our own curriculum reform efforts to illustrate this (and don't worry, we will provide more practical tips later in the chapter).

# BEGIN WITH THE END

Our program has been around for more than 60 years. We do some things extremely well, some things adequately, and a few things probably not so well (and are honest enough to say that). We knew we had room for improvement and updating, but we really wanted to ask the question of whether there were better ways to train our residents. We did not want to be complacent.

## "Operation Blow It Up"

Our small group of colleagues (the authors of this chapter) embarked on a mission of complete curriculum revision. We met monthly at lunch to discuss curricular reform for our general residency program. The program director invited a handful of seasoned clinician-educators to meet in an almost clandestine way, in what was playfully termed "Operation Blow It Up." We affectionately referred to it as "the OBIU meeting" or simply "OBIU." Our mission, as we accepted it, was to completely transform our entire residency training curriculum, broadly conceptualized at the beginning of this chapter, from orientation to graduation.

Much like a new psychotherapy case, we spent a few sessions gathering information. We listened to each other about what we liked or disliked about our curriculum, both experiential and didactic. We used the resident evaluations of our curriculum and discussed our own thoughts and experiences. One of our first action items was to gather a list of all of our graduates from the previous 17 years, a time period during which most of the OBIU group had been present. One member had not been present and provided a fresh perspective. We each reviewed the list and asked what characteristics of our graduates were most important to us and to our profession. We wanted to know if "the end product" we were producing was exactly what we wanted or if it needed further refining. This is very much in line with the concepts presented in the book *Understanding by Design* by Wiggins and McTighe (2005), although their focus was mainly on K–16 curriculum development, as well as Leadership Habit 2 as described by Covey (1989).

We began with the end. We determined that we appreciated graduates who put patients first, were empathic/compassionate, and had a fearless and natural curiosity and who had matured over their 4 years of training and become adept at complex medical decision making. We preferred graduates who had high initiative and worked well with others. We were also very interested, although not exclusively, in those who chose academic careers.

Based on these discussions, we made various and quick changes. We put even more emphasis on case conferences and clinical skills evaluations. We increased the frequency of case conferences and emphasized the generation of broader differential diagnoses. We increased the structure (higher and more standardized review criteria for faculty) and frequency (quarterly) of clinical skills verifications and put greater emphasis on the doctor–patient relationship and demonstration of empathy. We worked with the chair and hospital to bring in national-level trainers in trauma-informed care to further enhance compassionate care and help residents better understand the interplay of a patient's psychosocial and biological aspects.

Another change we made as a result of our work was to revamp our psychopharmacology curriculum (see "Tips for Curriculum Development" later). Our residents had performed well in this area on the Psychiatry Resident-In-Training Examination (PRITE) but had rated our psychopharmacology curriculum negatively. They were really telling us that they did not feel confident with their clinical knowledge, even if they could demonstrate it on a test.

We even discussed dress code and developed a small curriculum on it. This was not the most popular topic, but it certainly sparked a lot of discussion, and we have seen some changes. It is also a great way to incorporate discussions about professionalism and patient–physician relationships.

To encourage the development of academic careers, we incorporated more shared learning experiences, including conferences where faculty development and resident education coexisted. Topics included how to staff a clinic patient (from the attending and resident perspectives), suicide risk screening and assessment, and electronic medical record hand-off tools. The underlying theme was that we were a team that worked to accomplish the same goal. We have added "fireside chats" in which the program director and associate program directors meet monthly with individual postgraduate year (PGY) classes to discuss their questions and concerns and provide updates on the department to allow more transparency about how an academic department and practice functions.

Our program performed its ACGME self-study during the 2018–2019 academic year, so much of what we were doing during OBIU was pertinent. We were already thinking about where we wanted to be in 5 years and beyond. The ACGME self-study process and resources can help you structure your own OBIU as well; the following are some of the areas we examined during our OBIU/self-study process that we believe set the tone for our curriculum development and reform.

## What Are or Will Be the Strengths of the Program?

Despite the age of the program, it is important to pause and think about its *strengths* or aspirational strengths. Be very thoughtful and intentional about this in developing a curriculum in which residents will thrive. Begin with the end. For our program, we considered its top three strengths to be the richness of our substrate for clinical teaching, the program's "personality," and our learning climate.

In terms of our substrate for clinical teaching, residents got exposure to a wide range of patients:

- **Diagnostically:** *Full spectrum.* We were confident that our graduates, during their 4 years of training, saw it all, even very-low-prevalence diagnoses, and graduated with an exceptional level of confidence in managing common diagnoses.
- **Acuity:** *Full spectrum.* Residents used time-limited psychotherapy with patients who wanted to more fully actualize their potential, used electroconvulsive therapy with patients who had catatonia and were receiving tube feedings, and everything in between.
- **Patients requiring integrated care:** *Full spectrum.* On our psychiatric/medical inpatient unit, residents co-managed patients with the general internal medicine hospitalists who rounded daily on the unit, wrote notes and orders, and discussed patient care with the psychiatry team. Traditional consultations with the internal medicine, obstetrics and gynecology, and surgery specialties were available. On their movement disorder rotations, residents co-managed outpatients with neurologists, physical therapists, occupational therapists, stereotac-

tic neurosurgeons, advanced registered nurse practitioners, physician assistants, social workers, and neuropsychologists "embedded" in one neurological center. Residents got to see how each of these disciplines contributed to patients' overall quality of life and the bidirectional interactions between medical and psychiatric illness.
- **Complexity:** *Full spectrum.* Residents saw patients who were typical of those that a psychiatrist in private practice would see in a community population and were often their initial mental health professional. They served as a tertiary care provider for patients who had been seen by numerous prestigious medical centers and had sought us out because of ongoing diagnostic uncertainty, thus challenging the residents' interviewing skills and decision making regarding further workup. Some patients had been labeled "treatment resistant" or "refractory" and came to us for specialty services such as deep brain stimulation for OCD. Residents managed this range of patients.
- **Socioeconomic:** *Full spectrum.* Our 1,000-bed medical/surgical teaching hospital provides charity care for a huge population. Residents learned how resources were accessed for indigent patients on emergency and consultation-liaison rotations. They also provided almost all of the psychiatric care for the University of Florida faculty, staff, and their families.

## What Is the Personality of the Program?

Another important question we asked is, "What is the *personality* of the program?" Be very thoughtful about this; begin with the end. For us, we needed to know

1. Are these the type of faculty, residents, and staff that I would like to work and hang out with for the long haul?
2. Would they have my back if the occasion called for it?
3. Would I reach out to them for support if I needed to?

These questions are meant to get to the core of teamwork, professionalism, and leadership, all critical starting points for the success of any curriculum development.

## What Is the Learning Climate?

A major area that we wanted to evaluate was our *learning climate.* In our experience with many different learning climates, some were good fits and some were not. Good fits brought out our best, and learning soared. In poor-fit climates, learning seemed forced, and stress levels were way too high. Too much mental energy was siphoned off on being careful instead of fueling learning. Planning curriculum is a good time to pause and think about examples of each learning climate. Again, begin with the end.

### OPEN-DOOR POLICY

We have a fairly relaxed learning climate. Keep in mind that challenging and intense, hard work fit quite well into a relaxed learning climate. The ground in our department is pretty level. There are no "prima donnas" you have to tiptoe around. Faculty are amazingly approachable and accessible. We give residents our cellphone numbers and encourage them to call us. Office doors stay open; residents just sit down on the couch, and we stop whatever we are doing and try to help them. They do not have to go through anyone else to see us but simply call, text, email, or walk in and ask for help. Titles and seniority do not change faculty approachability or accessibility.

### THE 5-MINUTE RESIDENT INTERVENTION

Sometimes we cannot drop everything and give a resident uninterrupted open-ended time. They know this and do not expect us to fix their problem on the spot. What we do deliver on the spot can be accomplished in 5 minutes. This can be a powerful 5 minutes for them; they see us give them our full attention. For 5 minutes they are not competing with the grant or paper we have to get out the door today. They see us start from a position of "yes" and not from a position of "no." "Yes" to what? "Yes" to a solution that will only become apparent later, after we have carved out an hour of uninterrupted time for them. Being noticed—and we mean *really* noticed—in the distressed state they are in when they walk into our office can turn a 5-minute timeout for us into an amazing tonic of relief for them. There are no promises to solve anything in particular in that short time, but they come away with a plan. What plan can we come up with in 5 minutes? The plan—as explicit as though we signed a contract—is that we will apply our best thinking to help them when we learn more about their problem later. Imagine the curricular lesson of this and its application to patient and family care.

### IT'S OKAY TO SAY "I DON'T KNOW"

The next characteristic of our learning climate usually takes new interns a little time to trust. There is really nothing at stake when residents reveal to us that they do not know something. We do not think a knowledge deficit requires a negative or punitive response. Truly, the residents who do best in our program are usually fairly mature people who have good internal awareness of what they do and do not know and are transparent about this knowledge with faculty. We love when residents are transparent because it allows us to be strategic and focused with our teaching in order to shoot straight through the deficit. Residents who depend heavily on external quality control and need lots of monitoring or "exploratory surgery" to discover their knowledge deficits fit less well in our program.

## Sometimes It Is Necessary to Go Against the Grain

In today's psychiatric world, we must consider the relevance of teaching psychotherapy in psychiatric residency. Many of our graduates may not use some—or any—of these modalities directly in their future career, so why even teach them?

Psychiatrists are scientists of the psyche, and decision making and problem solving depend on the accurate collection of data from the patient. Without good data, one cannot make good clinical decisions. Patients' stories are complex, nuanced, and "hidden" from plain view. Our foundational belief is that psychotherapy provides a more complete understanding of the patient's history and symptoms so that we can make subsequent decisions and treatment plans, psychopharmacological as well as psychotherapeutic, more rationally and intentionally. In essence, to be a good psychopharmacologist, one must also be a good psychotherapist.

Inertia is often hard to overcome in curriculum design. One of us (G.L.K) had been out of academics for more than 30 years and decided to return for "the last third of his career" (we kid you not). He said, "I really want to start a psychodynamic psychotherapy clinic...that's my dream." Over the next year, he kept saying this over and over to the program director (J.A.H.), who one day finally said (in her most supportive manner) something like "So stop talking about it and just do it."

We have developed a separate, time-protected psychodynamic psychotherapy clinic. Residents in their third year work weekly with a minimum of two patients. The tenets of adult learning theory (see Chapter 1) involving the acquisition of knowledge, followed by supported problem solving and concluding with repeated practice, were instrumental in our structure for this clinic (VanLehn 1996). We began with weekly 2-hour sessions in July to introduce residents to psychodynamic psychotherapy, including watching videos and live therapy sessions. This was followed by 11 months of weekly 2-hour blocks of patient time in which residents managed psychodynamic psychotherapy cases and received short, real-time supervision and weekly asynchronous supervision with another supervisor.

In the third year of this clinic, we replaced the asynchronous supervision with a 45-minute small-group supervision lead-in. These group meetings explore clinical understanding and problem solving as they relate to a particular patient. The meetings are immediately followed by a 2-hour clinic block in which residents "practice" their newfound skills of psychodynamics, which are then briefly reviewed after the session. The group supervision/clinic is coupled closely with a weekly psychodynamic seminar that teaches multiple schools of psychodynamic theory and provides readings to reinforce what is learned. This clinic has been a significant boost to overall teaching, morale, and well-being. Residents get to know their patients better and have close supervision. Faculty have been energized to improve teaching and the clinic flow, creating constant and innovative curriculum development. The experience deepens residents' appreciation for patient complexity and the profundity of what it takes to change.

Many psychiatric residency programs include a third year of outpatient clinical experiences. In our clinic structure, the resident interviewed an established patient and immediately discussed that patient with an attending physician, ideally exploring diagnostic assessment and treatment plans through collaborative efforts. The resident and attending returned to the patient, discussed the plan, and discharged the patient, all within a 30-minute time frame. Problem solving and mentoring in this way were too rapid for any careful mastery and resulted in diagnostic imprecision and uncorrected heuristic errors. Residents felt pressured, anxious, and angry, with low levels of satisfaction and sense of self-competence. Informed again by learning theory (VanLehn 1996), we elected to "slow" the process down. The 30-minute return visit was extended to 45 minutes, which allowed longer consultations with the attending physician, immediate review of the literature, and more extensive treatment planning. The attending physician had more time to model techniques and interactions with the patient. This singular change contributed to better education and to the well-being of the resident, faculty, and patient.

Such "against the grain" ideas can be met with long looks from leadership and business managers that seem to ask, "You want to do what?" Our experience is that residents are completing their notes, phone calls, and other administrative work in the extra allotted time, which contributes to improved clinic quality metrics and fewer complaints of burnout. This outcome may help convince leadership that the financial disincentives are manageable. Sometimes you just need a nudge to get going.

Sometimes you just need to stop wishing and take the plunge. This can also go against the grain, but when you "begin with the end," you realize what is important and what you, as a training program, value.

# FROM "THE END" TO "THE PRACTICAL"

## Well, That's Fine for Your Program

We are a well-established program with years of experience, and we have a very good sense of our learning climate. If you are in a new program, you may feel as though you do not have this luxury. You are actually *lucky*! You can create the learning climate you want instead of trying to change a well-entrenched culture. You just have to have courage and take time to reflect about what it is you really want. You can do this. A good place to start is to utilize the tools of the ACGME Self-Study (see Table 11–1). Our OBIU model is in line with ACGME requirements because we focus on developing a certain type of graduate to fulfill institutional and community needs.

Many new program directors just want to know where to start with building a curriculum. They think, "lay the foundation and build up from there." This perspective makes intuitive sense and has merit. What we found in the OBIU process, however, was that knowing what you want your product—the end—to be and working backward is more rewarding. Starting from the ground up can get you lost in the weeds.

## Tips for Curriculum Development: Don't Reinvent the Wheel (If You Don't Have To)

Curriculum development is not a new endeavor. Many sage teachers have gone before you. A more recent review of didactic curriculum revision by Benson et al. (2018) can be instructive. They divided the curriculum into 20 overall content areas as guided by PRITE content (see Table 11–1) and the ACGME milestones:

1. Aging/Dementia
2. Approach to the patient
3. Cognitive-behavioral therapy
4. Child and adolescent psychiatry
5. Community psychiatry
6. Consultation-liaison/Emergency psychiatry
7. Health care policy
8. Law and psychiatry

9. Mood disorders
10. Neuroscience
11. Personality disorders
12. Psychodynamic psychotherapy
13. Psychopharmacology
14. Psychotic disorders
15. Quality and safety
16. Research literacy
17. Sociocultural psychiatry
18. Substance use disorders
19. Teaching/Career planning
20. Trauma-spectrum disorders

They reinforced the concept that curriculum development should not be the job of one person. Sexton et al. (2016) documented a different approach to psychiatry curriculum revision, which also focused on junior faculty development, that can be helpful.

The old saying of "don't reinvent the wheel" applies here. A great example of this is the psychopharmacology curriculum. The American Society of Clinical Psychopharmacology (see Table 11–1) has an extensive and complete psychopharmacology curriculum for residency training. For a relatively low cost, you can purchase and download premade PowerPoint presentations, and voilà! you have a curriculum. We incorporated this model curriculum into our didactic lecture series and have adapted it to our needs and supplemented when necessary for our goals.

Another way to develop curriculum is to adopt a favorite textbook (Table 11–2) in a needed topic area, such as interviewing skills, and develop teaching materials (e.g., slides, case discussions, handouts) from it. Then, just work your way through the textbook and included materials. If the textbook has 20 chapters, you have a minimum of 20 hours of teaching materials, and residents have 20 chapters of reading curriculum. One of our faculty members utilizes a textbook as the basis for his neuroscience lectures on mood disorders.

Another simple way to develop curriculum is to compile a group of journal articles on a given topic and develop discussion questions based on each article. For example, one might choose 5–10 articles on the subject of women's mental health, with an initial review article. Each article (or two) could be the subject of a 1- to 2-hour didactic session. A short (10-minute) lead-in didactic can be developed to explain the background and basic concepts, and then the paper (assigned in advance) could be discussed in a systematic way. An American Association of Directors of Psychiatry Residency Training (AADPRT) Model Curriculum has gone

**Table 11–2.** Some suggested textbooks and other books for resident teaching

| Title | Authors | General topic(s) |
|---|---|---|
| *Kaplan and Sadock's Synopsis of Psychiatry: Behavioral Sciences/Clinical Psychiatry*<br>Latest Edition: 11th (2015) | Benjamin J. Sadock, M.D., Virginia A. Sadock, M.D., and Pedro Ruiz, M.D. | General psychiatry |
| *Stahl's Essential Psychopharmacology*<br>Latest Edition: 4th (2008) | Stephen M. Stahl, M.D. | Psychopharmacology, neuroscience |
| *Depression and Bipolar Disorder: Stahl's Essential Psychopharmacology*<br>Latest Edition: 3rd (2008) | Stephen M. Stahl, M.D. | Mood disorders, psychopharmacology, neuroscience |
| *Handbook of Psychiatric Drug Therapy*<br>Latest Edition: 6th (2010) | Lawrence A. Labbate, M.D., Maurizio Fava, M.D., Jerrold F. Rosenbaum, M.D., and George W. Arana, M.D. | Psychopharmacology |
| *Psychiatry Test Preparation and Review Manual*<br>Latest Edition: 4th (2020) | J. Clive Spiegel, M.D., and John M. Kenny, M.D. | Board examination review |
| *Treatment Plans and Interventions for Depression and Anxiety Disorders*<br>Latest Edition: 2nd (2012) | Robert Leahy, Ph.D., Stephen Holland, Psy.D., and Lata McGinn, Ph.D. | Depression and anxiety treatment, psychotherapy |
| *Kaufman's Clinical Neurology for Psychiatrists*<br>Latest Edition: 8th (2017) | David Myland Kaufman, M.D., Howard L. Geyer, M.D., Ph.D., and Mark J. Milstein, M.D. | Clinical neurology |
| *Psychiatry and Clinical Neuroscience: A Primer*<br>Latest Edition: 1st (2011) | Charles F. Zorumski, M.D., and Eugene H. Rubin, M.D., Ph.D. | General psychiatry, clinical neuroscience |

**Table 11–2.** Some suggested textbooks and other books for resident teaching *(continued)*

| Title | Authors | General topic(s) |
|---|---|---|
| *The Dialectical Behavior Therapy Skills Workbook: Practical DBT Exercises for Learning Mindfulness, Interpersonal Effectiveness, Emotion Regulation, and Distress Tolerance*<br>Latest Edition: 2nd (2019) | Matthew McKay, Ph.D., Jeffrey C. Wood, Psy.D., and Jeffrey Brantley, M.D. | Dialectical behavior therapy |
| *Mind Over Mood: Change How You Feel by Changing the Way You Think*<br>Latest Edition: 2nd (2015) | Dennis Greenberger, Ph.D., and Christine A. Padesky, Ph.D. | Cognitive-behavioral therapy |
| *Neuroscience of Clinical Psychiatry: The Pathophysiology of Behavior and Mental Illness*<br>Latest Edition: 3rd (2018) | Edmund S. Higgins, M.D., and Mark S. George, M.D. | Neuroscience |
| *Treating Affect Phobia: A Manual for Short-Term Dynamic Psychotherapy*<br>Latest Edition: 1st (2003) | Leigh McCullough, Ph.D., Nathaniel S. Kuhn, M.D., Ph.D., Stuart Andrews, LMHC, NCC, Amelia Kaplan, Jonathan Wolf, and Cara Lanza Hurley | Psychotherapy |
| *The Psychoanalytic Model of the Mind*<br>Latest Edition: 1st (2015) | Elizabeth L. Auchincloss, M.D. | Psychoanalysis |
| *Psychiatric Interviewing: The Art of Understanding*<br>Latest Edition: 3rd (2017) | Shawn Christopher Shea, M.D. | Psychiatric interviewing skills |
| *Learning Psychotherapy: A Time-Efficient, Research-Based, and Outcome-Measured Psychotherapy Training Program*<br>Latest Edition: 2nd (2004) | Bernard D. Beitman, M.D., and Dongmei Yue, M.D. | Psychotherapy |

**Table 11–2.** Some suggested textbooks and other books for resident teaching *(continued)*

| Title | Authors | General topic(s) |
|---|---|---|
| *Massachusetts General Hospital Psychiatry Update and Board Preparation*<br>Latest Edition: 4th (2017) | Theodore A. Stern, M.D., John B. Herman, M.D., and David H. Rubin, M.D. | Board examination review |
| *Study Guide for the Psychiatry Board Examination*<br>Latest Edition: 1st (2016) | Philip R. Muskin, M.D., and Anna L. Dickerman, M.D. | Board examination review |
| *The Center Cannot Hold: My Journey Through Madness*<br>Latest Edition: 1st (2007) | Elyn R. Saks, M.D., J.D., Ph.D. | Schizophrenia |
| *Falling into the Fire: A Psychiatrist's Encounters with the Mind in Crisis*<br>Latest Edition: 1st (2013) | Christine Montross, M.D. | Patient encounters |

a step further and created a journal club curriculum. The National Neuroscience Curriculum Initiative has excellent learning modules for neuroscience that can be used directly or demonstrate different ways to break down topics with supplementary materials, including interactive and multimedia learning. The spectrum of topics to cover in a curriculum can be gleaned from various readily available sources. We also recommend the American Board of Psychiatry and Neurology (ABPN) content blueprint not only for PGY4 board review courses but also for overall didactic curriculum development. Sexton et al. (2016) used the ACGME competencies and requirements and the ABPN and PRITE content outlines. They also reviewed model curricula published in academic journals, AADPRT, and MedEdPortal (see Table 11–1).

## When You Do Have to Start From Scratch

When content areas are new or very specific to your training program (e.g., mental health laws in your particular state), we advise you to start small. Develop one lecture in the area, revise it based on feedback, and, if necessary, develop a next-step lecture or learning activity (discussion based or journal club). Take it one step at a time. The AADPRT Curriculum Committee offers tips on how to develop a curriculum (see Table 11–1) as well as many peer-reviewed curricula available for direct use, adaptation, and examples to guide your own curriculum development. There are examples of small (one or two lectures) and large (complete coverage of topic) curricula; for example, 1-, 3-, and 4-year curricula/outlines are available for addiction psychiatry, cultural psychiatry, child and adolescent psychiatry, evidence-based medicine, professionalism and ethics, psychiatric interviewing, and quality improvement. Other topics include the history of psychiatry, integrated/collaborative care, systems-based practice, and consultation-liaison psychiatry.

## You *Can* Teach What You Don't Know

You may be asked to teach things you do not know well or at all. One of us (J.A.H.) started a women's mental health clinic and curriculum several years ago with very little prior knowledge or practical experience. A couple of residents asked to start the clinic, and it can be difficult to say no to enthusiastic residents who are interested in doing important work. Reading textbooks and chapters, review articles, and primary source journal articles increased her expertise until she became the go-to faculty member for this area. It takes courage to learn and teach something you do not already know, but it can be done. Be brave and step outside your comfort zone.

## Curriculum Development Does Not Rest Solely on the Program Director's Shoulders: You Are Not Alone

The entire faculty, including the chair, is responsible for the training program and curriculum. ACGME program requirements for faculty state that core faculty should play a significant role in developing and providing or presenting the curriculum. Do not hesitate to require teaching faculty assistance and participation. Junior faculty must be involved in teaching to develop their skills and prepare their portfolio for promotion.

It is human to feel daunted by these responsibilities. Remember to network and talk with other program directors, associate directors, and training faculty. Program directors and faculty in other specialties can help in areas that fall under the common program requirements (e.g., quality improvement and scholarly activity). A good working relationship with the neurology and internal, family, and emergency medicine program directors and faculty may also help with cross-development of curricula. Subspecialty program directors, when available, can collaborate closely with you to develop and provide curricula for your program.

The AADPRT and other organizations listed in Table 11–1 have mentoring programs, listservs, and annual meetings that offer opportunities for fruitful learning and exchange of ideas around curriculum development. Advocate for yourself with your chair or division chief to join professional organizations and to attend meetings focused on teaching. By going to education-related conferences, you will learn that you are not alone. When it comes to curriculum development, everyone is in the same proverbial boat.

## — KEY POINTS —

- Think broadly and beyond the classroom about curriculum.
- Begin with the end for curriculum development: what should residents learn, and who do you want them to be when they leave your program?
- Don't reinvent the wheel. Borrow liberally from previously developed curricula, but give credit where due.
- Start small, one lecture at a time, to build the curriculum.
- Don't be afraid to go against the grain and beyond the status quo in your program, department, or field.
- Branch out and learn to teach something new.

- Don't go it alone. Enlist the help of your chair and teaching faculty, including junior faculty, and network both within and outside your institution.

# REFERENCES

Benson NM, Puckett JA, Chaukos DC, et al: Curriculum overhaul in psychiatric residency: an innovative approach to revising the didactic lecture series. Acad Psychiatry 42:258–261, 2018

Covey SR: Begin with the end in mind: principles of personal leadership, in The 7 Habits of Highly Effective People: Restoring the Character Ethic. New York, Simon and Schuster, 1989, pp 95–144

Sexton JM, Lord JA, Brenner CJ, et al: Peer mentoring process for psychiatry curriculum revision: lessons learned from the "mod squad." Acad Psychiatry 40:436–440, 2016

VanLehn K: Cognitive skill acquisition. Annu Rev Psychol 47:513–539, 1996

Wiggins G, McTighe J: Understanding by Design, 2nd Edition. Alexandria, VA, Association for Supervision and Curriculum Development, 2005

## CHAPTER 12

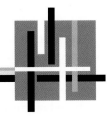

# ACCREDITATION, FINANCING, AND RESIDENCY ADMINISTRATION

Randon S. Welton, M.D.

**Psychiatrists** become residency program directors for a variety of reasons, but rarely out of a love for administrative detail. Awareness of these details, however, is essential for the success of the program and the director. The program director becomes the default expert in financing the residency, recruiting and selecting residents, maintaining accreditation, administering the residency program, preparing residents for board certification, and interacting with various agencies that impact residency education. This chapter gives an overview of some of the most important rules and regulations and how to find and keep current about those that impact residency training.

## FINANCING THE RESIDENCY

Most of the funding for graduate medical education (GME) comes from the Centers for Medicare and Medicaid Services through Medicare. In

2013, Medicare spent more than $11 billion on GME (Schuster 2017). Medicare supports GME through direct and indirect payments to residency training sites (e.g., hospitals), not to the residency itself. Direct medical education payments are intended to pay the salaries of residents and supervising physicians and to defray some of the administrative costs of training programs (e.g., accreditation fees). Payments are based on the number of residents working at the site. Until 1997, hospitals could expand their revenue by adding residents to existing programs with Accreditation Council for Graduate Medical Education (ACGME) approval. The 1997 Balanced Budget Act placed a limit ("cap") on the number of Medicare-supported residency slots. The cap was determined by the number of residents working at any given site in 1996 and has remained in place ever since, with limited exceptions (Dower 2012; Mihalich-Levin and Cohen 2015; Rich et al. 2002). Indirect medical education payments subsidize hospitals for other expenses associated with training residents and have historically accounted for as much as two-thirds of the total Medicare funding for GME (Schuster 2017). These payments exist because care in hospitals with GME programs is more expensive. Training hospitals are often tertiary referral centers and see patients with more complex illnesses who often need specialist care and receive more laboratory and ancillary studies. Lengths of stay increase when residents care for patients. Indirect payments offset these "hidden costs" of GME and are based on the number of residents working at the site and the turnover of inpatient beds (Dower 2012; Mihalich-Levin and Cohen 2015; Rich et al. 2002).

Numerous complaints exist about Medicare funding of GME. Organizations such as the Institute of Medicine have recommended significant changes in how training is funded. Resident caps are now more than two decades old and do not consider current physician workforce needs. The calculations that determine funding are based on inpatient services with an implicit, currently erroneous assumption that most training and patient care happen with inpatients and thus do not account for contemporary care models. Medicare payment formulas lead to significant discrepancies in funding. For example, in 2012, teaching hospitals in New York received an average of $131,000 per resident, whereas those in Texas received only $61,000 (Iglehart 2015). The future of federal Medicare funds for GME remains uncertain and tied to congressional action.

Another major source of federal support for GME comes through the U.S. Department of Veterans Affairs (VA). The VA began supporting GME after World War II and is now the largest provider of health care training in the United States. In 2017, more than 43,000 residents received at least some of their training at a VA site. The VA participates in more than 2,600 GME programs in 83 different types of specialty training (Chang and Brannen 2015; Office of Academic Affiliations 2019). As well as providing training sites, by 2014 the VA funded more than 10,000 resident positions. The Veterans' Access to Care through Choice, Accountability, and Transparency Act of 2014 called for a further increase of 1,500 funded positions, primarily in primary care and mental health specialties (Chang and Brannen 2015). In 2018, the VA paid out more than $1.75 billion to support GME (Heisler and Panangala 2018), but few residents supported by VA funding have the VA as a sponsoring institution. The vast majority of VA-funded residents are part of affiliation agreements between the VA and a separate sponsoring institution. The VA reimburses the sponsoring institution for the cost of resident salaries and benefits while they are working at a VA site and allows faculty members time to train and supervise residents. It also pays the additional costs associated with supporting teaching units (Schuster 2017).

Another source of residency funding is Medicaid. As of 2016, 42 states and the District of Columbia contributed $4.26 billion to medical education through state-controlled Medicaid funds. The majority of this was through managed-care contracts, with the remainder being in fee-for-service payments (Schuster 2017).

Three U.S. Department of Defense (DoD) armed services—the army, navy, and air force—sponsor GME programs, both in stand-alone training programs and in locations where they contribute residents to a civilian training program. In 2015, it was estimated that the DoD supported more than 1,800 residents in 109 specialties (Schuster 2017).

The Health Resources and Services Administration provides funding via three additional federal programs. Since 1999, the Children's Hospital GME (CHGME) payment program has supported resident training in children's hospitals. The 2016 budget for this program was $295 million. The Affordable Care Act created a Teaching Health Center GME program to expand opportunities for primary care residents in community-based ambulatory settings. The future of this program remains unclear because in 2017, the cost of this program was more than $157,000 per resident. The Title VII Health Professions program is designed to address the shortage of rural and inner-city health care providers; these funds support the additional cost of training residents in an ambulatory environment with uninsured patient populations (Schuster 2017).

Health care systems may choose to pay directly for GME and then be reimbursed by billing insurance companies for the care provided by trainees in conjunction with faculty members. Such billing may only occur when residents have an active state medical license and is usually possible only in those specialties where reimbursement sufficiently covers training expenses. If residents are part of a health care system's preferred provider network, the cost of the training is offset by the savings inherent in having the residents provide care rather than the more expensive community providers. It is difficult to estimate the number of residents trained in this fashion (Schuster 2017).

## RECRUITING AND SELECTING RESIDENTS

Most residency programs acquire new residents through the National Resident Matching Program (NRMP), which runs "the Match," a legally binding algorithm that sorts through applicant and program preferences. Residencies may choose not to participate in the Match and reach out to applicants directly to offer training contracts, but relatively few psychiatry programs do so. Full participation with the Match is necessary to use the resources of the NRMP and the Electronic Residency Application Service (ERAS), which is administered by the Association of American Medical Colleges. Not participating greatly limits the amount of information available about applicants.

The NRMP has an "all-in policy" that requires participating programs to use the Match for all of their first-year resident slots (National Resident Matching Program 2019a). Programs may apply for exceptions to this policy, but these are more likely to be granted to programs in rural or medically underserved areas or to those participating in Rural Scholars, Family Medicine Accelerated Track, and Innovative Programs. Active-duty military residents are assigned to residencies through a separate DoD process. In residencies with both military and civilian residents, the military residents are assigned through the DoD, and civilian residents are typically selected through the Match (National Resident Matching Program 2019a).

The NRMP's "Match Participation Agreement for Applicants and Programs" fully describes the NRMP process and typically has minor changes from year to year. It defines the eligibility of applicants, discusses the roles of the applicants and training programs, and specifies the dates and timing of the application and selection process. Applicants select residency programs and send applications through ERAS. Residency programs use ERAS to review applications, which include a Medical Student Performance Evaluation (MSPE; also known as a dean's letter), medical school transcript, a personal statement, U.S. Medical Licensing Examination/Comprehensive Osteopathic Medical Licensing Examination scores, and letters of recommendation. Applicants attest to whether they are able to meet the physical and mental requirements of residency training, if they experienced any delays in training, or if they have had any significant legal problems. Programs choose applicants to invite for an interview and then create a rank order list (ROL) of the most desired applicants. Applicants make a parallel ROL of their most-desired programs (National Resident Matching Program 2019c).

Program directors are responsible for ensuring that all current residents and faculty maintain the highest ethical standards during the interview, ranking, and matching process. These standards exist because of prior instances of programs pressuring applicants to commit to positions in ways that disadvantaged the students. Some of the more challenging NRMP rules limit communication between representatives of the residency program and applicants. Certain lines of questioning are strictly forbidden. For example, current rules specify that during the entire interview and Match process, programs may not ask applicants the names, specialties, geographical location, or other identifying information about other residency programs to which they have applied (National Resident Matching Program 2019c). Federal antidiscrimination laws prohibit questions about an applicant's age, gender, religion, sexual orientation, and marital/family status. Programs may express an interest in the candidate but may not ask the candidate about his or her intention to rank the program. Program directors are discouraged from "unnecessary" postinterview communication and in particular must not solicit or require further information once the interview is completed, because applicants often perceive these postinterview requests as coercive. Programs must avoid even the appearance of attempting to influence an applicant's ranking preferences (National Resident Matching Program 2019b). Although the rules seem straightforward, they appear to be violated frequently. Many of the 6,700 candidates surveyed after the 2015 Match listed potential violations of Match communication policies. Most applicants (72%) had been asked at least once about their interview experiences at other programs. Thirty-eight percent had been asked about their marital status and 15% had been asked directly how highly they would rank the program. Twenty-two percent of women had been asked about children or plans to have children. Postinterview communication occurred in 91% of the applicants surveyed, generally in the form of a thank you card or email initiated by the applicant, reportedly sent out of fear that not sending one would lower a program's ranking of the applicant. Other studies have indicated similarly high rates of potentially forbidden questions during interviews (Berriochoa et al. 2018).

The NRMP dictates the Match schedule and announces it yearly. Programs receive applications in mid-September, and the MSPEs become available in early October. Program directors usually send out official invitations to interview between October and January. Programs generally interview between 8 and 10 candidates for every available position. In January, the program must officially declare the number of positions they will be filling for the next academic year. Both programs and applicants submit their ROLs to the NRMP by mid-February (National Resident Matching Program 2019c). The NRMP computer algorithm starts with applicants' preferences and then considers residency preferences to optimize placement of applicants. Unmatched applicants may participate in the Supplemental Offer and Acceptance Program, whereby they are informed which residency programs have openings and can apply to one of those programs (National Resident Matching Program 2019c). This process is explained further in Chapter 9. The NRMP changes yearly, so familiarizing yourself with current rules is critical.

# MAINTAINING ACCREDITATION

## Accreditation Council for Graduate Medical Education

The ACGME is the principal organization responsible for the accreditation of medical and surgical residencies in the United States. It also serves as the parent organization for the Residency Review Committee (RRC) and the Clinical Learning Environment Review (CLER). These integrated organizations create and monitor conditions and requirements for residency training. Psychiatric program directors must be extremely familiar with the most current ACGME Common Program Requirements (CPR) and Psychiatry Requirements. These guidelines cover almost all aspects of psychiatry training and are updated regularly. The ACGME website (www.acgme.org) provides the most current information to guide you in managing your program.

## Common Program Requirements

The CPR prescribe the educational experiences, knowledge, skills, attitudes, and resources that are mandated for residency training across all specialties (Accreditation Council for Graduate Medical Education 2020b). The goal of the CPR is to ensure an environment that fosters the development of physicians who are models of clinical excellence, compassion, professionalism, and scholarship. The requirements specify that programs have in place institutional agreements that formalize responsibility for teaching, supervising, and evaluating residents at different sites.

The CPR list the basic requirements for program directors, including the qualifications, responsibilities, and specific resources that they must have, and describe other requirements for training, including a program coordinator, faculty members, and space and learning resources for trainees. On the trainee side, the CPR define which candidates are eligible for GME and defines six general competencies that provide the foundation for instructing, evaluating, and promoting residents. Scholarly activity among residents and faculty is another requirement. The CPR have recently included requirements on patient safety, quality improvement, supervision, learning environment, and wellness.

#### *PATIENT SAFETY*

The ACGME has paid increased attention to patient safety. Residents, faculty, training programs, and health care organizations must promote patient safety and understand and report near misses and adverse clinical events. Residents and faculty members must receive feedback about the events they report. Residents should understand the benefits and procedures of formal patient safety activities, such as root cause analysis and morbidity and mortality conferences, and should participate in real or simulated interprofessional clinical safety activities.

#### *QUALITY IMPROVEMENT*

Interdisciplinary quality improvement projects, including projects related to reducing health care disparity, are required. Programs must ensure residents receive instruction on designing and completing such projects. To encourage quality improvement, residents and faculty members must receive data on the quality metrics and benchmarks related to their patient populations.

#### *SUPERVISION*

The ACGME requires that supervision be structured, deliberate, and progressive. Patients under the care of a resident must have an identifiable, appropriately credentialed/privileged attending physician who is ultimately responsible for their care. Residents must inform patients of their dual roles as trainee and care provider. Residency programs must have a consistent method to increase residents' responsibility and authority. The CPR describe specific levels of training and supervision.

#### *LEARNING ENVIRONMENT*

The CPR discuss the learning and work environments in great detail, similar to the CLER (see next section). The ACGME highlights the environment as a joint responsibility shared by the sponsoring institution, the clinical training sites, and the residency program.

*WELLNESS*

Both the CPR and CLER emphasize faculty and resident wellness. Residency programs, in partnership with their sponsoring institutions and clinical training sites, are obligated to address workplace safety, work intensity, and other factors that might impact resident well-being. Residents and faculty must have opportunities to attend medical and mental health appointments during working hours and have access to screening for burnout, depression, and substance use disorders. Programs must also continue to emphasize identifying and mitigating fatigue. One major ACGME initiative to combat fatigue was the restriction of duty hours (Accreditation Council for Graduate Medical Education 2020b). The CPR restrict the number of consecutive hours a resident can work in a patient care role, set out the hours required between shifts, and address moonlighting experiences, in-house call, and limitations to night float rotations (Accreditation Council for Graduate Medical Education 2020a). Some educators continue to express concerns that duty-hour restrictions diminish the quality of training; a multispecialty study of 464 program directors in 2011 reported that most thought the duty-hour limitations decreased resident continuity with hospitalized patients and would not decrease resident fatigue. Many also thought the restrictions would decrease their ability to ensure residents' proficiency in the core competencies (Antiel et al. 2011).

## Clinical Learning Environment Review

Beginning in 2012, the ACGME extended its regulatory purview to hospitals, medical centers, and ambulatory-care practices where residents and fellows train by establishing mandatory CLER visits. The findings of these visits are intended to improve the quality and safety of education and patient care and are not intended to be used for accreditation of sponsoring institutions or residency programs. The CLER program was designed to provide formative feedback to leaders at clinical training sites and sponsoring institutions regarding six areas of focus: patient safety, health care quality, care transitions, supervision, duty hours and fatigue management and mitigation, and professionalism (Weiss et al. 2014). "Health care quality" includes promoting efforts to decrease health care disparities in society and formal training in cultural competency. The supervision standards require that physicians and nurses have an efficient way to determine which procedures residents may perform independently and which require supervision. "Care transitions" standards involve developing formal supervised processes for patient handoffs.

During a CLER visit site, inspectors meet separately with leaders from the sponsoring institution and the clinical site, program directors, faculty members, and residents and speak at random with other staff members (Wagner et al. 2016b; Weiss et al. 2014). Site visitors provide an immediate debriefing and then a follow-up letter. CLER proposes a revisit every 24 months to monitor progress and improvements. The ACGME released results from the first round of CLER visits with nearly 300 institutions in 2016. These results substantiated the concerns that instituted the CLER process. Although residents frequently reported potential patient safety concerns, fewer than half had received follow-up after their report. In most clinical sites (59%), few residents and fellows were familiar with basic quality improvement concepts, and in more than half of the clinical sites, residents categorized their training in cultural competency as largely generic. Most residents had no objective way of knowing whether fellow residents were competent to perform procedures without supervision. One in six reported that at some point in training they had been pressured to compromise their integrity to satisfy the demands of an authority figure (Wagner et al. 2016a). Findings such as these led to more standardized trainings for residencies and standardized processes within hospitals.

In 2018, after visiting many locations a second time, CLER released another set of findings. Some slight improvement was found in "professionalism," however, fewer residents were participating in interprofessional patient safety investigations, and many still had not received feedback after reporting patient safety concerns. The CLER report expressed disappointment in the lack of alignment between residents' quality improvement projects and the stated priorities of the workplace. Standardized, supervised transitions of care had declined. Many residents still reported being placed in or witnessing a situation in which supervision was inadequate. Despite continuing efforts to inform residents about the dangers of practicing medicine while fatigued, the percentage who reported caring for patients while fatigued increased (Koh et al. 2018). Efforts continue to integrate the CPR with CLER standards.

## ACGME Program Requirements for Psychiatry Residencies

The RRC takes the CPR and adapts them for specific specialties. The requirements are divided into *core* and *detail*. Core requirements define the structure and resources for residency training and must be demonstrated in every residency. Some variability is allowed in detail requirements, which generally describe structures or processes that help meet the core requirements. Programs may use alternative or innovative approaches to meet the intent of the detail requirements. The requirements define the competencies to be addressed, clinical experiences that must be present, and the particular committees, administrative structure, and reporting requirements of the ACGME (Accreditation Council for Graduate Medical Education 2020a). Because the document that defines psychiatric residency training changes frequently, we recommend that you obtain the most recent iteration of the requirements.

### Accreditation Data System

The RRC tracks residency programs through an internet-based accreditation data system called WebADS. WebADS allows the RRC to closely follow changes within residencies and to monitor their performance and compliance with ACGME requirements, including new CPR and CLER initiatives. Again, because this is an ever-moving target, we refer you to WebADS to determine what is required in terms of documentation at the yearly update.

## PREPARING RESIDENTS FOR BOARD CERTIFICATION

### American Board of Psychiatry and Neurology

The American Board of Psychiatry and Neurology (ABPN) oversees the process to obtain and maintain board certification. The ABPN adds few additional requirements to residency administration. Training directors must confirm training experiences as required by the internet-based precertification information management system. ABPN presently requires that the resident pass at least three clinical skills verification (CSV) examinations that are conducted by a board-certified psychiatrist trained to perform the CSV and are meant to certify basic competency in three areas: clinical interview, mental status examination, and presentation. The timing, format, and requirements for examiners and grading are available on the ABPN (www.abpn.com) and American Association of Directors of Psychiatric Residency Training (www.aadprt.org) websites.

## IMPLEMENTING THE REQUIREMENTS

Implementation of such a wide variety of requirements involves continual negotiation with the department, sponsoring institution, and clinical sites.

## Department

The program director must have a close working relationship with departmental leadership and the department chair. The program director works with the chair or vice chair for education to manage faculty appointments, evaluations, and feedback. Budget and staffing are typically the chair's prerogative. Chairs must support their program director's protected time to design and administer the residency. They can be program directors' greatest ally or obstacle, and this relationship warrants considerable investment.

## Sponsoring Institution

According to the ACGME, "The Sponsoring Institution is the organization or entity that assumes the ultimate financial and academic responsibility for a program of graduate medical education, consistent with the ACGME Institutional Requirements" (Accreditation Council for Graduate Medical Education 2020a). Because they often oversee many different residency and fellowship programs, sponsoring institutions set institution-wide policies, implement and monitor individual residency compliance with ACGME policies, and select and approve the appointment of program directors. The CLER and CPR standards underscore the importance of sponsoring institutions working with residency programs and training sites to promote patient safety, health care quality, care transitions, supervision, duty hours/fatigue management and mitigation, and professionalism. The due process for residencies regarding resident academic/behavioral probation or termination must be coordinated with the sponsoring institution.

## Clinical Sites

Often the biggest challenge for program directors is balancing education with patient care. Residents are often seen as a less expensive means to meet the health care organization's priority: providing high-quality care for patients while remaining financially viable. They may, therefore, push for a maximum amount of resident time. The demand for residents to provide patient care may imperil the educational value of the experience. Careful and specific negotiations should occur before residents are assigned to a site, including the number of residents, maximum patient load, night/weekend/holiday coverage, and protected time for education. These will need to be reviewed periodically.

Resident time is usually measured as full-time equivalents (FTEs), wherein 1 FTE equals 40–50 hours of clinical care per week. For health care organizations, however, paying eight resident salaries does not equate to eight FTEs of resident clinical time in their facility. Didactics, supervision, and other mandatory educational activities also come from the time paid for by the organization. They must accept that residents are less efficient than faculty members and will see fewer patients per hour. With the presence of residents, faculty members assume the role of supervisors, which makes them less efficient as well. Observing residents, discussing patient interactions, reviewing documentation, and making suggestions for changes in management all take time. Faculty members will also be asked to work with residents on quality improvement, patient safety, and research projects. These are also time consuming. In an organization that previously focused exclusively on patient care, this is a change in culture. The residency program director should explain the long-term value of a training program. Time spent working with residents may be recouped in increased faculty satisfaction, recruitment, and retention. Resident-led quality improvement projects can improve the efficiency and patients' experience of medical care. Finally, patient safety activities can lead to better outcomes for patients.

# CONCLUSION

The administrative and regulatory demands of running a residency program are numerous. Monitoring ACGME requirements and trying to implement them in a way that is both financially and practically viable and improves the educational culture may challenge the most creative program director. Awareness of and active engagement with the various agencies and regulations that govern the professional life of program directors allows us to do the thing we really value: training the next generation of psychiatrists.

## — KEY POINTS —

- Program directors must understand the role of the Centers for Medicare and Medicaid Services and other agencies in funding residency programs.
- The yearly acquisition of residents is typically through the National Residency Matching Program (NRMP), whose regulations must be understood and followed by program directors.
- The program director is responsible for ensuring that faculty and residents abide by NRMP policies throughout the interview and Match process.

- The Accreditation Council for Graduate Medical Education (ACGME) oversees all aspects of residency training and is the parent organization for the Residency Review Committee and the Clinical Learning Environment Review.
- The ACGME is working to integrate standards for patient safety, health care quality, care transitions, supervision, duty hours and fatigue management and mitigation, and professionalism among residency programs, sponsoring institutions, and clinical training sites.
- The Residency Review Committee tracks programs' compliance with ACGME requirements through the yearly internet-based accreditation data system WebADS.
- Program directors interact with the American Board of Psychiatry and Neurology through its precertification website to ensure that graduates are prepared to take their board certification examinations.
- Program directors must work closely with department leadership, sponsoring institutions, and clinical training site leadership to ensure that residents' experience remains focused on their education in addition to providing high-quality care for their patients.

# REFERENCES

Accreditation Council for Graduate Medical Education: ACGME Program Requirements for Graduate Medical Education in Psychiatry. Chicago, IL, Accreditation Council on Graduate Medical Education, 2020a. Available at: https://www.acgme.org/Portals/0/PFAssets/ProgramRequirements/400_Psychiatry_2020.pdf. Accessed November 18, 2020.

Accreditation Council for Graduate Medical Education: ACGME Common Program Requirements (Residency). Chicago, IL, Accreditation Council on Graduate Medical Education, 2020b. Available at: https://www.acgme.org/Portals/0/PFAssets/ProgramRequirements/CPRResidency2020.pdf. Accessed November 18, 2020.

Antiel RM, Thompson SM, Hafferty FW, et al: Duty hour recommendations and implications for meeting the ACGME core competencies: views of residency directors. Mayo Clin Proc 86:185–191, 2011

Berriochoa C, Reddy CA, Dorsey S, et al: The residency match: interview experiences, postinterview communication, and associated distress. J Grad Med Educ 10:403–408, 2018

Chang BK, Brannen JL: The veterans access, choice, and accountability act of 2014: examining graduate medical education enhancement in the Department of Veterans Affairs. Acad Med 90:1196–1198, 2015

Dower C: Health policy brief: graduate medical education. Health Affairs, August 16, 2012, pp 1–4

Heisler EJ, Panangala SV: The Veterans Health Administration and medical education: in brief, in Congressional Research Services, February 13, 2018. Available at: https://fas.org/sgp/crs/misc/R43587.pdf. Accessed August 9, 2019.

Iglehart JK: Institute of Medicine report on GME: a call for reform. N Engl J Med 372:376–381, 2015

Koh NJ, Wagner R, Newton RC, et al: The CLER national report of findings 2018: trends in the CLER focus areas. J Grad Med Educ 10(4 suppl):69–76, 2018

Mihalich-Levin L, Cohen A: Demystifying what Medicare GME payments cover and how they're calculated. Acad Med 90(9):1286, 2015

National Residency Matching Program: All-in Policy: Main Residency Match. NRMP website, 2019a. Available at: http://www.nrmp.org/all-in-policy/main-residency-match. Accessed August 16, 2019.

National Residency Matching Program: Match Communication Code of Conduct. NRMP website, 2019b. Available at: http://www.nrmp.org/communication-code-of-conduct. Accessed August 16, 2019.

National Residency Matching Program: Match Participation Agreement for Applicants and Programs. Washington, DC, National Residency Matching Program, 2019c. Available at: https://mk0nrmp3oyqui6wqfm.kinstacdn.com/wp-content/uploads/2018/09/2019-MPA-Main-Residency-Match_Applicants-and-Programs.pdf. Accessed August 16, 2019.

Office of Academic Affiliations: Medical and Dental Education Program (website). U.S. Department of Veterans Affairs, 2019. Available at: https://www.va.gov/oaa/GME_default.asp. Accessed August 16, 2019.

Rich EC, Liebow M, Srinivasan M, et al: Medicare financing of graduate medical education. J Gen Intern Med 17:283–292, 2002

Schuster BL: Funding of graduate medical education in a market-based healthcare system. Am J Med Sci 353(2):119–125, 2017

Wagner R, Koh NJ, Patow C, et al: Detailed findings from the CLER national report of findings 2016. J Grad Med Educ 8(2 suppl 1):35–54, 2016a

Wagner R, Patow C, Newton R, et al: The overview of the CLER program: CLER national report of findings 2016. J Grad Med Educ 8(suppl 1):11–13, 2016b

Weiss KB, Bagian JP, Wagner R, Nasca TJ: Introducing the CLER pathways to excellence: a new way of viewing clinical learning environments. J Grad Med Educ 6:608–609, 2014

# CHAPTER 13

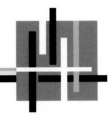

# EVALUATION OF RESIDENT TRAINEES

Kim-Lan Czelusta, M.D.

**Management** of residents with problems and problem residents is one of the most time-consuming yet important responsibilities of the residency program director. Addressing resident difficulties in a meaningful and timely manner is paramount. Complex and often conflicting issues related to fairness to the resident, the program, and the public require a clear process in place, not only to support both the program director and the resident but also to promote the best outcome possible.

In addition to the work of residency recruitment, program directors have a critical role in helping trainees successfully complete residency training. Trainees often have difficulty during these formative years of professional development. Some difficulties are straightforward and can be easily addressed, whereas others may be extremely challenging, time consuming, and stressful to all involved. Residents' status as both an employee and a trainee simultaneously guides and complicates the process of addressing problems. Unlike traditional employer or supervisory situations in which the accommodations made are usually related

Acknowledgments: Kathy Sanders, M.D., and James Lomax, M.D.

to disability, program directors make numerous training accommodations to support struggling trainees toward successful graduation. Such modifications may include changing rotations or call schedules, increasing supervision, decreasing workload, or having a trainee repeat a clinical experience for remediation. When approaching a resident's difficulty, residency directors must balance three essential tenets—1) fairness to the resident, 2) safety of the public, and 3) adherence to program policies—with the goal of helping that resident successfully complete residency training.

Every program director should have a systematic algorithm for addressing resident difficulties. Consulting the chief residents and clinical competency committees, associate program directors, vice chair for education, and department chair are often initial steps. Depending on the severity of the concern, an early discussion with the designated institutional official (DIO) and the general counsel is also wise. Throughout, the program director must ensure adequate documentation with evaluation data and meeting notes because such documentation will be critical if formal disciplinary action is needed.

## EARLY DETECTION OF RESIDENT DIFFICULTIES

Program directors should have multiple sources of information to help identify problems, particularly as new residents are adjusting to the rigors of training. Sources of data may include attending supervisors, chief residents, site directors, service chiefs, supervising on-call faculty, resident peers, administrative staff, patients, nurses, or other hospital staff. If the concern is minor and is not representative of a pattern, the program director will need to decide whether the issue warrants direct intervention or if an early intervention with a chief resident, attending, or assistant program director would be sufficient and more tolerable for the resident. Interpersonal or communication concerns involving resident peers may be best addressed by the chief resident; similar concerns involving clinical staff may be best addressed by the attending supervisor. Regardless of who initially contacts the resident, documentation of the concern and subsequent intervention is important in case the concern is the beginning of a pattern. Resident challenges can often be associated with one or more ACGME competencies. Table 13–1 provides common resident difficulties, categorized by core competencies.

**Table 13–1.** Common resident difficulties based on core competencies

| Core competency | Examples of resident difficulty |
|---|---|
| Patient care | Patient complaints (also interpersonal and communication skills) |
| | Inadequate safety assessments (also medical knowledge) |
| | Incomplete differential diagnoses (also medical knowledge) |
| | Disorganized psychiatric formulations |
| | Poor clinical decisions (also medical knowledge) |
| Medical knowledge | Failing clinical skills verifications |
| | Low scores on in-service examinations |
| | Failing U.S. Medical Licensing Examination Step 3 |
| Practice-based learning and improvement | Failure to use current evidence in decision making |
| Interpersonal and communication skills | Interpersonal conflict with patients, peers, staff, or health care team |
| | Inappropriate comments in work environment (also professionalism) |
| | Ineffective communications with patients (also professionalism) |
| Professionalism | Timeliness for work, pages, call, or documentation (also interpersonal and communication skills) |
| | Intoxication at work |
| | Poor attendance at required educational activities |
| | Failure to notify team/program when out ill (also interpersonal and communication skills) |
| System-based practice | Failure to involve appropriate agencies and referrals (also interpersonal and communication skills) |
| | Recommendations not compatible with community resources |

# DIFFERENTIAL CONSIDERATIONS

Multiple factors contribute to problems with resident performance, not all of which can be influenced by the program director. For instance, if the concern is a result of family or personal stressors (e.g., financial problems, marital tensions, illness, family conflict), the program director may offer emotional support and refer the resident to the institution's employee assistance program (EAP) or mental health service. The program director may consider temporarily reducing the resident's workload to allow more time to address the situation but must balance how long such a modified, reduced schedule is reasonable while still ensuring that the resident meets expectations for graduation. If the resident's difficulty is a result of problems on a clinical unit or team, then the program director may help elucidate and address any contributing external factors. For instance, if the problem stems from a specific staff member who has had similar past behavior, the program director can help loop feedback to the clinical supervisor, who can then intervene with the problematic staff member. Residents who reflect and receive support after the program director presents concerns may improve their performance with no other intervention, depending on their responsiveness to feedback. If other team members contribute significantly to the resident's difficulty, the attending physician or service chief may need to become involved. Sometimes, difficulties with team members may be a result of incompatible interpersonal styles.

Most residents have a predictable developmental course during residency, but some struggle more than others during the transition from medical student to resident. Increased patient care responsibilities, combined with administrative tasks, new electronic medical records (EMRs), teaching expectations, and development of more advanced specialty-specific clinical skills, may be overwhelming and result in difficulties, including problems managing time. These transition difficulties may be worsened if the medical school that the resident attended had a particularly different culture. For instance, a resident from a smaller school may thrive in a single hospital system with one EMR but struggle in a program with multiple affiliated hospitals that use different EMRs. In addition, geographical transitions can be jarring—relocating from a familiar environment with established sources of support to a new area with limited supports can be isolating and stressful, exacerbating the stress of training. Goodness of fit with the residency program may contribute to a difficult adjustment and, if severely incompatible, may necessitate transfer. Geography, program size, number of clinical sites and faculty, program culture, patient volume, typical work hours, and call type and frequency all contribute to "fit." Incompatible specialty choice may also produce resident difficulties.

Finally, resident psychopathology or medical illness can play a significant role in difficulties. Referral for treatment to the institution's psychiatric counseling service or EAP or to a community provider may help the program director determine how best to support the resident or to provide independent support to the resident. Some residents may not feel comfortable seeing a mental health provider who is employed at the same institution due to confidentiality concerns, despite Health Insurance Portability and Accountability Act (HIPAA) safeguards. In addition, if the clinician is a former supervisor or a faculty member who may be placed in an evaluator role for the resident in the future, these conflict-of-interest scenarios may be additional barriers to treatment. Thus, it is important to have multiple treatment-provider options available and to openly address any resident trepidation. A medical leave of absence or withdrawal from the program, depending on the severity of the problem, may be necessary to allow the resident time to address personal health needs. Residents who have limited insight or are noncompliant with treatment recommendations are at particular risk for the need for time away from the program. Many residents worry about the potential impact a leave of absence may have on future reporting requirements for credentialing and licensure. Thus, familiarity with these requirements is essential when counseling the resident about next steps.

## POSSIBLE INTERVENTIONS FOR RESIDENTS WHO ARE HAVING DIFFICULTY

Policies and procedures for residents with difficulties vary among institutions and state boards and should be followed carefully by program directors. The following are some suggested frameworks to intervene.

### "Cup of Coffee" Meeting

The first meeting to address a nascent or mild concern may be informal, with the goal of informing the resident about the concern (Hickson et al. 2007); it must be in private and may be initiated and led by a program director's designee, such as the assistant program director or chief resident. Regardless of who leads the meeting, the feedback must be specific, with expectations clearly communicated to minimize ambiguity. A follow-up meeting 1–2 weeks later may help support the resident after he or she has had time to process and reflect. Sample isolated concerns that could be addressed with an initial casual meeting include 1) showing up late for call shifts, 2) unprofessional comments during resident meetings, 3) reports of inappropriately describing patients during rounds, or 4) repeated late documentation.

## Written Improvement Plan or Remediation

If informal interventions are insufficient to improve behavior or the concern is more serious, a formal written improvement plan with clearly delineated expectations may be warranted. The program director will need to obtain specific and detailed feedback from those reporting the concerning behavior. If the source of feedback is a fellow trainee or other learner, confidentiality may need to be protected. Repeating a rotation or period of training may be an option for residents who do not successfully meet the expectations of a specific clinical experience. Program directors must be aware of the state licensing board reporting requirements for remediation or other formal adverse actions and notify the resident if the state medical board requires mandatory reporting. Directors should be well versed in disciplinary options in the institutional graduate medical education policy. Consulting the institution's legal counsel and DIO for guidance is highly recommended, especially for program directors who are dealing with resident concerns for the first time. For an initial concern that does not warrant more serious disciplinary action, many program directors work with residents to identify opportunities to improve without employing an intervention that would impact the residents' career and result in mandatory, perpetual reporting whenever they apply for medical licensure or hospital privileges. Improvement plans must spell out the expectations as well as the subsequent steps, such as probation or another reportable disciplinary action, should the problematic behavior not improve or worsen. Concerns that could warrant a more formal improvement plan include repeated lateness or unapproved absences, frequent interpersonal conflicts with coworkers, missing required didactics, and unprofessional behavior with team members.

## Probation

Probation is rarely an initial step unless the resident problem is significant. Most state medical licensing boards list probation as a reporting requirement for program directors, so any residency program will need to note this disciplinary action on malpractice insurance applications and credentialing and licensure documents when requested on behalf of the resident. Resident peers and even faculty are often affected by and aware of problems of such severity well before the program director. Due to the confidential nature of disciplinary actions, fellow residents' responses can vary; some may assume the program director is not doing enough to address the resident with problems, whereas others may view the intervention as too harsh. This latter scenario is more likely to occur if the resident having difficulty is sharing his or her experience with peers while the program director is respecting confidentiality.

Most programs have due-process procedures that allow residents to appeal disciplinary actions, so sufficient data about the resident's difficulties as well as institutional support from the DIO and legal counsel are necessary before taking any action that mandates reporting or could be appealed. The appeals process causes undue stress on the resident with problems and on the program director as well as on other residents, who may experience a combination of reactions such as anxiety, anger, relief, tension, and sadness.

## Nonrenewal or Termination of Employment Contract

When probation does not result in improvement or the problem is sufficiently severe, either nonrenewal or termination of the resident's contract may be necessary. Program directors do not make these decisions without careful review, deliberation, and consultation. If termination is being considered during the latter part of the academic year, the director may have the option to not renew the residency contract. In this scenario, the institution or employer must give the resident a minimum period of notice, often 3–4 months, as contractually specified. This period allows the resident to pursue transfer to another program and allows the program director to fill the residency slot. Decisions to prevent a resident from continuing or completing training are often made when the risk for the institution and the public outweigh the resident's goal of completing training. The program director will also need to develop consistent communication regarding the resident's departure for future inquiries. Consultation with the chair, DIO, and institutional general counsel is recommended regarding any future written or verbal communication about the resident's performance and any credit to be given. A resident's early departure from a training program leaves the program director to manage the reactions of other residents and faculty without being able to share specific details. Directors should use this opportunity to review the program and institution's policies for addressing concerns and supporting residents with difficulties. Providing a forum for residents to ask general questions can help quell their angst. Ideally, program directors review information about difficulties with residents at the start of training, before specific problems actually occur.

## UNINTENDED CONSEQUENCES FOR OTHER CONSTITUENTS

Although program directors may spend countless hours ensuring that a resident problem is handled in a thoughtful, methodical, and fair manner, managing its effects on other residents, faculty, and clinical sites cannot be ignored. If a resident with problems is unable to perform previously scheduled responsibilities or departs early, the program director often must rely on the remaining team members and clinical site to develop an alternative plan to ensure patient care and that other residents' training experiences are not adversely disrupted. Inevitably, the affected members of the team will work more than anticipated, so ensuring compliance with duty hours and adequate learning environments for remaining residents will be essential. The program director may need to address faculty responses as well, which may vary from relief to anger. Returning the focus to patient care and residency education can often assuage tensions.

## TWO EXAMPLES

### John: Inefficiency and Poor Clinical Judgment

John is a new intern at a large training program that has multiple clinical sites, each with a different EMR. Prior to residency training, John grew up and attended college and medical school in his hometown. He maintained close relationships with numerous childhood friends and lived at home with his tight-knit family until residency. John was excited about matching into a large residency program in a new city, but his excitement diminished quickly. He got along well with his resident peers but missed his longtime friends and the daily comforts of family and social support. John was also adjusting to living independently for the first time while balancing his new role as an employee. He quickly became overwhelmed. Attending supervisors noted both his strong work ethic and his inefficiency on evaluations, including his willingness and frequent need to stay later than his peers to complete patient care responsibilities. Chief residents reported that John got along well with the team and was a contributory team member.

During their first semiannual meeting, John and the program director reviewed his evaluations together. John was disappointed that his evaluations were barely above average; he felt especially bad about comments that his inefficiency occasionally delayed treatment planning. He resolved to become more efficient and acknowledged that he was having a harder transition to residency than he had expected. He appreciated the program director's encouragement, support, and suggestion to use the available psychiatric counseling service. A few months later, the director received an evaluation from the attending physician in the psychiatry emergency department with concerns about John's inefficiency and "barely average" performance. The attending specifically noted delays in patient treatment caused by John's need for more workup time compared with his peers. In addition, his treatment plans for patients were not thorough and deemed subpar.

The program director contacted the attending physician to request more details about John's performance. The attending stated that although John "passed" the rotation, he was a "weak" resident who may have more trouble as expectations and level of independence increase. Both the attending physician and the program director were particularly concerned about John's upcoming, required emergency department night float rotation during his second postgraduate year. The attending, like others, noted John's strong work ethic and advocacy for patients as strengths. Although John was initially both surprised and embarrassed about this feedback, he was eventually appreciative of the program director's customized learning plan to help him succeed. The plan included identifying a faculty mentor—a prior attending physician who recognized John's strengths of patient advocacy and his work ethic. The mentor agreed to adjust the faculty call schedule to match his own schedule with John's so he could work directly with John in the emergency department, where John's weaknesses were most notable. In addition, the mentor worked with John on strategies to improve efficiency with EMR templates and practiced more focused interviewing with him to improve his initial assessments.

Over time, John's confidence increased, and he was able to develop more comprehensive patient treatment plans and to complete his EMR documentation in a timely manner. He was no longer listed as "delinquent" for EMR deadlines. The program director checked in with John and his mentor monthly, and by the next Clinical Competence Committee review, the committee members and program director unanimously agreed that the learning plan had been successful. This proactive approach by the program director and a faculty mentor who was willing to go above and beyond for a resident avoided the need for more formal action requiring reporting to outside agencies.

Several key factors in the program director's approach helped this resident improve and achieve success:

1. **Identification of a faculty mentor:** The program director was able to collaborate with a specific willing faculty mentor who could adjust the schedule and work directly with the struggling resident in the setting where his weaknesses were most readily revealed.

2. **Collaboration with clinical site:** The program director worked with the clinical site's service chief to discern specific weaknesses. Then the director, the chief of psychiatry, and the designated faculty mentor worked together toward a learning plan for the resident.
3. **Targeted skills training to improve specific deficiencies:** The faculty mentor worked with the resident to specifically focus on his key weaknesses.

## Jennifer: Repeated Tardiness and Other Professionalism Concerns

During her first 2 years of residency, Jennifer's attendance at didactics was intermittently in the lower range compared with her peers but not low enough to warrant intervention beyond a warning during semiannual evaluation reviews, when her low attendance was flagged. In her third postgraduate year, however, two outpatient clinic attending physicians reported Jennifer to the program director for periodic lateness that had resulted in patient complaints and concerns related to clinic flow. The director reviewed these concerns with Jennifer, and her tardiness improved temporarily. During her group therapy rotation, however, Jennifer was absent as group leader, and the attending co-leader scheduled a meeting to address her unapproved and unscheduled absence. Jennifer apologized for her absence and explained that her alarm did not go off that morning. The attending physician made the program director aware of Jennifer's absence and subsequent explanation.

A few months later, the director received a call from another attending physician who shared concerns about Jennifer's rigidity, specifically noting her resistance to modifying a treatment plan after discussion with her attending physician. The program director met again with Jennifer to review this new feedback about her interpersonal interactions. Jennifer explained that she was having difficulty waking up in time for work in the morning and eventually acknowledged that she was struggling with substance use. The program director gave Jennifer referrals to the institution's psychiatric counseling service as well as the EAP.

A couple of weeks later, Jennifer requested a medical leave of absence. Jennifer's peers were notified that she was on medical leave, and the call schedule was adjusted. During the third week of her medical leave, Jennifer submitted a resignation letter, explaining that she needed to leave the city to distance herself from triggers that exacerbated her substance misuse. The program director reviewed Jennifer's training situation with the institution's legal counsel and DIO and then scheduled a meeting with Jennifer to review the verification of training letter they would provide for her on request after she left the program to ensure all were aware of the content of future communications.

When the program director notified the residents that Jennifer was not returning, they had a broad spectrum of reactions and responses. Some who had covered for her lapses in work responsibilities thought the director had waited too long to address concerns. Others were angry about covering more call shifts for the remainder of training now that Jennifer had resigned. Some residents expressed anxiety that they too could "get in trouble" and not complete training, and others felt sad and worried about Jennifer. The program director could not disclose specific details about Jennifer's situation other than making the notifications about her medical leave and resignation.

Given the residents' strong and mixed responses, the program director's team scheduled multiple group meetings with individual classes, as well as individual residents on request, to discuss resources to help struggling residents as well as general processes related to residency disciplinary action. They were transparent about not being able to reveal specific information about specific residents due to privacy concerns but welcomed questions, including hypothetical ones, that residents had. In addition, the team met with chief residents to offer support because many residents had turned to their chiefs to vent and share concerns.

Approximately 2 years later, Jennifer contacted the program director to request a letter of reference as she reapplied to psychiatry residency programs closer to her hometown, where she had been living and had extensive family support.

Key factors in this case include

1. **Feedback:** Program directors depend on early and specific feedback about resident concerns.
2. **Management and support of other residents:** Periodic review of supportive resources, as well as due process for resident problems, is essential. Residents' perception of a program director's intervention may nonetheless vary from premature to insufficient.
3. **Clarification of future correspondence:** Departing residents will need a verification of training letter. This should be reviewed with the DIO, general counsel, and the resident to ensure everyone is aware of the letter's content.

## — KEY POINTS —

- Most residents have a predictable developmental course during residency training, but some may struggle during the transition from medical student to resident.
- In approaching a resident difficulty, the residency director is continually balancing 1) fairness to the resident, 2) safety to the public, and 3) adherence to program policies.
- Early intervention by the program director can minimize adverse effects on not only the struggling resident but also resident peers and clinical services.

- A systematic algorithm for addressing resident difficulties is essential and should include consultation with the designated institutional official and general counsel.
- Common modifications to help struggling residents include changing rotations or call schedules, increasing supervision, decreasing workload, or repeating a clinical experience.
- Policies and procedures for residents vary among institutions, and state medical boards have different reporting requirements. Awareness of policy, procedure, and reporting requirements is critical to adequately address a resident concern.
- Program directors often manage faculty reactions, especially if a struggling resident prematurely leaves the training program.
- For residents who receive formal disciplinary actions or who do not successfully complete the residency program, the program director should finalize a verification of training letter and share that letter with the resident to minimize future misunderstanding.

## REFERENCE

Hickson GB, Pichert JW, Webb LE, et al: A complementary approach to promoting professionalism: identifying, measuring, and addressing unprofessional behaviors. Acad Med 82(11):1040–1048, 2007

## CHAPTER 14

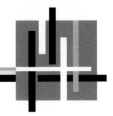

# SUBSPECIALTY TRAINING IN PSYCHIATRY

William Newman, M.D.
John Hearn, M.D.
Anne McBride, M.D.
Carrie Ernst, M.D.
Anna Kerlek, M.D.

> Choose a job you love, and you will never have to work a day in your life.
>
> Anonymous

**Psychiatric** subspecialties provide a mechanism for psychiatrists to pursue specialized training in defined areas of psychiatry. Fellowship program directors and faculty who share their passion for a subspecialty with their trainees may kindle an early interest that helps drive the decision to pursue a career in psychiatry or psychiatric subspecialties.

# HISTORY OF PSYCHIATRY SUBSPECIALTY ACCREDITATION

Despite a general trend toward medical subspecialization in the United States in the past century, the American Board of Psychiatry and Neurology (ABPN) has remained relatively conservative with developing new subspecialties (Faulkner et al. 2011). The ABPN offered its first subspecialty certificate, in child psychiatry, in 1959; they did not approve another until geriatric psychiatry in 1991. Since then, the ABPN has added certifications in addiction psychiatry (1993), forensic psychiatry (1994), and consultation-liaison psychiatry (2005).

The ABPN also recognizes several interdisciplinary subspecialties available to psychiatrists, including pain medicine (2000), sleep medicine (2007), hospice and palliative medicine (2008), and brain injury medicine (2011). In the initial "grandfathering" period, candidates could receive credentialing based on their clinical experience; subsequently, all candidates for certification were required to complete an Accreditation Council for Graduate Medical Education (ACGME)-accredited fellowship.

The process for ABPN approval of a subspecialty is complex. Leaders from subspecialty organizations request new certifications (Juul et al. 2004). The ABPN evaluates whether the proposed subspecialty would dilute the general field and whether the function could otherwise be met by general psychiatrists. Then, if appropriate, the ABPN submits the proposal to the American Board of Medical Specialties (ABMS). The ABMS reviews proposals for subspecialties in committee and submits them to voting representatives for approval. Following ABMS approval, the Residency Review Committee (RRC) for psychiatry develops training criteria for ACGME review and accreditation and subsequently reviews individual training programs in the subspecialty (Juul et al. 2004).

Several subspecialty proposals did not receive approval, including administrative psychiatry, adolescent psychiatry, and psychoanalysis. A proposal for consultation-liaison psychiatry was initially rejected but later approved as psychosomatic medicine. In 2018, the official name was changed back to consultation-liaison psychiatry in response to concerns that the term "psychosomatic medicine" was problematic.

# CURRENT ACGME FELLOWSHIPS

The ACGME currently accredits nine psychiatric subspecialty programs (Table 14–1). Psychiatry residents may also pursue non-ACGME accredited fellowships, such as public and community psychiatry, women's mental health, behavioral neurology/neuropsychiatry, and integrated care. Many of these specialized fields have their own professional societies or may be included as components of recognized fellowship programs, but they are not recognized as subspecialties by the ABPN.

Despite recent increases in applications to general psychiatry residency programs, application to most psychiatry fellowship programs has plateaued or, in some cases, declined (Agapoff and Olson 2019). Although the total number of psychiatry residents increased from 5,176 in the 2014–2015 academic year to 6,247 in the 2018–2019 academic year (20.7% increase over 5 years), the total number of consultation-liaison and geriatric psychiatry fellows decreased over this same 5-year period (Accreditation Council for Graduate Medical Education 2019b). Forensic, child and adolescent, and addiction psychiatry have fared better, with either a stable number or a net increase in the number of fellows (Table 14–2).

Although precise public data are lacking, we can estimate fill rates using graduate medical education (GME) census track data for the projected number of year-1 positions (Brotheron and Etzel 2018) and ACGME data for the actual number of first-year fellows (Accreditation Council for Graduate Medical Education 2019b) (Table 14–3). For example, fewer than half of available geriatric psychiatry fellowships were filled between 2006 and 2016 (Kirwin et al. 2016). National Resident Matching Program (NRMP) data show improved fill rates for the subspecialties of child and adolescent psychiatry (72.8%–83.7%) and consultation-liaison psychiatry (61.9%–68.9%) in 2019 compared with 2018 (National Resident Matching Program 2018, 2019). Some positions may also be filled outside the NRMP. Many consider this to be a burgeoning public health crisis involving too few psychiatric subspecialists to meet the growing clinical demands of subspecialty populations, such as children, individuals with substance use disorders, and the elderly (Agapoff and Olson 2019; Dean 2017).

## General Information for Fellowship Applicants

Interested applicants can familiarize themselves with subspecialty fields and fellowship training opportunities in many ways, such as reaching out to faculty within their institution, community psychiatrists, or faculty at other institutions. In some cases, a potential applicant might do a visiting elective rotation. Resident membership in a relevant national subspecialty organization (Table 14–4) offers opportunities to attend annual meetings and to network with current trainees and fellowship direc-

**Table 14–1.** Accreditation Council for Graduate Medical Education–accredited subspecialty programs available to psychiatrists

| Specialty | Length, *years* | Number of programs (2019–2020)[a] | Areas of focus |
|---|---|---|---|
| Addiction medicine (multidisciplinary) | 1 | 57 | Prevention, evaluation, diagnosis, treatment, long-term monitoring, and recovery of individuals with substance use disorders or unhealthy substance use and of those with substance-related health conditions |
| Addiction psychiatry | 1 | 50 | Prevention, identification, and treatment of individuals with substance use and co-occurring mental health disorders, including subpopulations such as pregnant women and individuals with HIV or hepatitis C; training occurs in a variety of settings, such as opioid treatment programs and residential treatment programs |
| Brain injury medicine (physical medicine and rehabilitation) | 1 | 21 | Prevention, diagnosis, treatment, and management of medical, physical, psychosocial, and vocational problems in individuals with brain injury from trauma, stroke, neoplasm, anoxia, and other brain disorders |
| Child and adolescent psychiatry | 2[b] | 139 | Evaluation, diagnosis, and treatment of disorders of thinking, feeling, or behavior in children and adolescents and their families (American Academy of Child and Adolescent Psychiatry 2019); training encompasses the full range of human development |

**Table 14–1.** Accreditation Council for Graduate Medical Education–accredited subspecialty programs available to psychiatrists *(continued)*

| Specialty | Length, *years* | Number of programs (2019–2020)[a] | Areas of focus |
|---|---|---|---|
| Consultation-liaison psychiatry | 1 | 61 | Assessment and treatment of behavioral/psychiatric symptoms in patients with medical and surgical problems in both inpatient and outpatient medical, surgical, and obstetrical settings; diagnosis and treatment of psychiatric disorders in medically ill patients, understanding the relationship between medical, neurological, and psychiatric conditions and treatments, and appreciating how psychological factors affect physical conditions |
| Forensic psychiatry | 1 | 48 | Clinical practice, education, and research into the ways that legal issues and psychiatry overlap; may include assessment and treatment of individuals involved in the criminal or juvenile justice systems and performing formal risk assessments; fellowship training includes clinical work in correctional settings, state hospitals, and community settings, training on testifying at trials, and scholarly activities (Kelly et al. 2017) |
| Geriatric psychiatry | 1 | 60 | Care of older adults with complex neuropsychiatric disorders that occur later in life, such as mild neurocognitive disorder with behavioral symptoms, late-life depression, and phase-of-life problems; fellows train in various settings, including long-term care facilities, geriatric psychiatry inpatient units and outpatient clinics, and cognitive disorders assessment services (Tampi et al. 2019) |

**Table 14–1.** Accreditation Council for Graduate Medical Education–accredited subspecialty programs available to psychiatrists *(continued)*

| Specialty | Length, *years* | Number of programs (2019–2020)[a] | Areas of focus |
|---|---|---|---|
| Hospice and palliative medicine (multidisciplinary) | 1 | 154 | Improving a patient's quality of life and decreasing suffering by managing physical, psychological, social, and spiritual needs of patients and their families in the setting of a serious illness, including during the end of life |
| Sleep medicine (multidisciplinary) | 1 | 85 | Multidisciplinary specialty focused on the assessment, monitoring, treatment, and prevention of sleep disorders utilizing medications, clinical evaluation, physiological testing, and imaging |

[a]Accreditation Council for Graduate Medical Education 2019c.
[b]This is a 2-year program that can be started after 3 or 4 years of general psychiatry residency training.

**Table 14–2.** Number of active fellows by specialty or subspecialty and academic year: 2014–2015 to 2018–2019

| Program | 2014–2015 | 2015–2016 | 2016–2017 | 2017–2018 | 2018–2019 | 5-year change |
|---|---|---|---|---|---|---|
| Psychiatry | 5,176 | 5,358 | 5,616 | 5,907 | 6,247 | +20.7% |
| Child and adolescent | 820 | 826 | 840 | 865 | 869 | +6.0% |
| Consultation-liaison | 82 | 79 | 80 | 86 | 71 | −13.4% |
| Forensic | 66 | 72 | 63 | 79 | 66 | 0% |
| Addiction | 66 | 80 | 77 | 74 | 83 | +25.8% |
| Geriatric | 58 | 58 | 56 | 53 | 52 | −10.3% |

*Source.* Accreditation Council for Graduate Medical Education 2019b.

**Table 14–3.** Estimated fill rates for psychiatry fellowship program year-1 positions, 2018–2019

| Specialty | Total projected year-1 positions,* *N* | Estimated fill rate,* % | NRMP fill rate 2018, % | NRMP fill rate 2019, % |
|---|---|---|---|---|
| Child and adolescent | 494 | 90 | 72.75 | 83.7 |
| Consultation-liaison | 124 | 57.3 | 61.9 | 68.9 |
| Forensic | 109 | 60.6 | N/A | N/A |
| Addiction | 111 | 72 | N/A | N/A |
| Geriatric | 123 | 42.3 | N/A | N/A |

NRMP=National Resident Matching Program.
*2018–2019.
*Source.* Accreditation Council for Graduate Medical Education 2019b; Brotheron and Etzel 2018; National Resident Matching Program 2019.

tors. Many organizations have "how to" guides for applying. In addition to program listings on subspecialty organization websites, the ACGME website (www.acgme.org) and Fellowships and Residency Interactive Database (www.ama-assn.org/residents-students/match/freida) offer up-to-date information on training programs.

**Table 14–4.** National (U.S.) psychiatric subspecialty organizations

| Subspecialty | National organization | Website |
|---|---|---|
| Child and adolescent | American Academy of Child and Adolescent Psychiatry | www.aacap.org |
| Consultation-liaison | Academy of Consultation-Liaison Psychiatry | www.clpsychiatry.org |
| Forensic | American Academy of Psychiatry and the Law | www.aapl.org |
| Addiction | American Academy of Addiction Psychiatry | www.aaap.org |
| Geriatrics | American Association for Geriatric Psychiatry | www.aagponline.org |

## Application Process

The timeline and process for fellowship application depends on the subspecialty. The NRMP oversees the Match for child and adolescent and consultation-liaison fellowships. Applicants must register for the Match in the fall of the year prior to the anticipated fellowship start date. Program lists are finalized in December, with Match results released in early January. Most NRMP-participating fellowships accept applications after July 1 for entry in the following year and interview applicants between July and early December. Some child and adolescent programs offer early positions outside of the Match. Residents can apply to child and adolescent fellowship positions at the end of either postgraduate year (PGY) 2 or PGY3. Fellowship programs that do not use the NRMP often accept applications in the spring of the year prior to starting fellowship (middle to end of PGY3 year), interviewing and offering positions on a rolling basis.

Since 2013, child and adolescent psychiatry applicants must apply through the Association of American Medical Colleges' Electronic Residency Application Service (ERAS). Other psychiatric subspecialties do not use the ERAS, so each program has its own application requirements, and interested residents must contact individual programs for information about their application process. Programs generally request the applicant's curriculum vitae, a personal statement, and two or three letters of recommendation. Most consultation-liaison psychiatry programs use an application created by the Academy of Consultation-Liaison Psychiatry. Forensic psychiatry programs typically require a writing sample, ideally related to a forensic experience.

### Information for International Medical Graduates

Many psychiatric subspecialty fellowship programs welcome international medical graduates (IMGs). Programs vary in their visa requirements and sponsored categories. Historically, only physicians who had completed a general psychiatry training program accredited by the ACGME or the Royal College of Physicians and Surgeons of Canada were eligible for appointment to an ACGME-accredited psychiatry subspecialty fellowship. In July 2019, however, the ACGME changed the Common Program Requirements for 1-year fellowships (Accreditation Council for Graduate Medical Education 2019a), allowing IMGs from residency programs with ACGME International Advanced Specialty Accreditation to apply for U.S. fellowships. These requirements may change over time, so we suggest referring to the ACGME website.

## BENEFITS OF SUBSPECIALTY TRAINING

### Fostering Interest

The pursuit of subspecialty training generally requires a high degree of passion or interest in the selected field in order to balance the expense of training. In addition to the application process during general psychiatry residency and the extra years of training, most subspecialists must complete another expensive and time-consuming board examination as well as general psychiatry boards. Subspecialty association membership dues, continuing medical education, and maintenance of certification for two board certifications add to the cost.

Another factor contributing to lower matriculation into subspecialties is that many medical students or general psychiatry residents have broad interests and a lack of exposure to subspecialty fields. To increase subspecialty exposure, students may participate in subspecialty clerkships or elective months. Formal programs, such as the Klingenstein Third Generation Foundation (www.ktgf.org), fund programs at select institutions to expose medical students to child and adolescent psychiatry. Additional resources or scholarships to attend annual conferences, receive mentorship, and pursue interests through professional organizations may enhance trainee exposure.

General psychiatry residents may also benefit from earlier subspecialty exposure than the typical required experience in order to develop their interest and establish specialized mentors. The fourth year of residency often is the only time to pursue electives but may be too late to inspire residents to pursue subspecialty training in time to apply. For example, applications for child and adolescent psychiatry fellowships are accepted soon after the start of the third academic year of general psychiatry for those who "fast track." General programs that provide child psychiatry experiences during the third year provide significantly less opportunity to foster interest in the field. Alternatively, some general programs create early interest tracks so that residents have more opportunities to explore such interests.

## Combining Subspecialty Interests

Trainees may wish to combine their subspecialty interests. For example, child forensic psychiatrists have unique expertise regarding juvenile justice and civil litigation. Geriatric forensic psychiatrists better provide guidance and care for the aging incarcerated population. Adolescent addiction psychiatrists can provide developmentally appropriate care for a population that requires critical intervention. Highly subspecialized psychiatrists may more easily establish career niches. Additional training and expertise may also expedite opportunities for promotion in academic settings.

## Standard of Care and Practicing Outside of Scope

Although subspecialty training better prepares physicians to provide the highest-caliber care to specific populations, there are not enough fellowship-trained psychiatrists available to adequately serve each unique population. In fact, primary care physicians frequently provide mental health treatment. In 2010, 20% of primary care office visits in the United States were for mental health (Cherry and Schappert 2014). Primary care physicians often become the primary manager of psychiatric disorders due to lack of access to outpatient mental health services (American Academy of Family Physicians 2018). In many places, general psychiatrists are the sole practitioners available to treat all mental health needs due to lack of subspecialty access options.

Physicians have an ethical obligation to provide appropriate patient care. The American Medical Association Code of Ethics instructs physicians to "provide care for patients with difficult to manage medical conditions" (American Medical Association Council on Ethical and Judicial Affairs 2017). The code specifies, however, that physicians "practice at their full capacity, but not beyond." Physicians must ensure that they practice above the standard of care, which includes practicing within their established scope of practice. Although general psychiatrists commonly incorporate aspects of psychiatric subspecialties, it is unlikely that doing so currently constitutes practicing outside of their scopes of practice. However, as psychiatric subspecialties expand both the relevant knowledge base and further differentiate themselves, general psychiatrists will need to pay close attention to this issue.

General psychiatry residents are exposed to some aspects of subspecialty training. The ACGME Program Requirements currently specify that general residents receive 2 months of experience in child and adolescent psychiatry as well as consultation-liaison psychiatry, 1 month of both geriatric psychiatry and addiction psychiatry, and experience in forensic psychiatry. Similarly, the ABPN board certification in psychiatry includes examination in multiple subspecialty domains.

Professional subspecialty organizations often develop guides and practice parameters that are relevant to the specialized field. Although these are not meant to necessarily represent the standard of care, such guides typically provide recommendations for practice based on reviews of the relevant literature and expert consensus and may help the generalist providing subspecialty care.

## SUBSPECIALTY WELLNESS

There is some attention in the literature to improving wellness in general psychiatry trainees (Bentley et al. 2018; Kang et al. 2019), but very little information in the literature addresses issues specific to the psychiatric subspecialties.

Each psychiatric subspecialty faces unique challenges to wellness. Child and adolescent psychiatrists often discuss physical, sexual, and emotional trauma experiences with the most vulnerable patients and families. Forensic psychiatrists are routinely exposed to details of horrific traumas during both criminal and civil evaluations. Consultation-liaison psychiatrists often become involved in cases involving ethical dilemmas, unrealistic patient or family requests, or disagreements between clinical services about treatment and disposition planning. Addiction psychiatrists feel added pressure from the national attention to the "opioid epidemic" and the stigma attached to substance use disorders. Geriatric psychiatrists frequently face end-of-life care, with attendant ethical issues and family conflicts. Attention needs to be paid to these subspecialty-specific challenges and their potential effects on the wellness of both subspecialists and general psychiatrists.

The potential benefits of subspecialty training are a notable offset to these issues. Monotony can contribute to burnout in general psychiatry practitioners. Subspecialty training allows practitioners to diversify their practice and maintain professional fulfillment. Teaching in fellowship programs may additionally maintain job satisfaction.

# RECRUITMENT INTO FELLOWSHIP PROGRAMS

## Differences From General Psychiatry Residency Recruitment

General psychiatry residency programs are highly competitive. Most fellowships, however, are in a "buyer's market," which necessitates attention to recruitment. Although often less formal, fellowship interviews require careful attention to detail. Providing interview schedules in advance helps applicants feel prepared for the experience. The interview day is often the primary mechanism for advertising the strengths and special features of the program. Polished print or online materials, meals, and direct personalized contact with the program director are all critical.

## General Approaches to the Interview Day

Program strengths are not always obvious to applicants. It is therefore important to highlight strengths when promoting your program nationally at meetings and with colleagues, on department websites, and when interviewing. Faculty and administrative staff should feature examples of innovative educational experiences and clinical programs during recruitment. Consider the "program's portfolio" and use a biopsychosocial approach to feature aspects of the program (Waheed et al. 2019).

## Timeline for Fellowship Recruitment

Effective recruitment requires strategic planning and commitment. Visibility, influence, and mentoring are paramount. Because many trainees become interested in career options during medical school, subspecialist presentations at medical student interest group meetings can be useful. Shadowing clinicians or rotations in longitudinal clinics may pique student interest, as may hosting lunches about "hot topics" in psychiatric subspecialty practice.

Clerkship experiences should include some type of subspecialty exposure, from placement on a specialty unit to small-group discussions or lectures. Electives during the fourth year and in early residency create excitement about fellowships. Subspecialty faculty must provide lectures and become involved in the residency interview process, attend and provide grand rounds, and participate in departmental committees to increase interest. The more subspecialties are integrated into a department, the more likely trainees will see them as career options.

## Recruitment Challenges

The average starting age of new psychiatry residents was 30.4 years in 2018 (Accreditation Council for Graduate Medical Education 2019b). At graduation, when deciding on their next steps, residents may have other considerations, such as a partner, children, or aging family members. Fellowship applicants also have potential jobs offering much higher salaries in general psychiatry.

Subspecialty training does not guarantee a higher salary. Data from 2017 reveal that the academic child and adolescent psychiatrist mean and median total compensations/salaries are now less than those of academic general psychiatrists in all areas of the country. Among all psychiatrists, child and adolescent psychiatrist mean and median salaries remain below those of general psychiatrist counterparts in the East and South and remain comparable in the Midwest and West. Information from other subspecialties in psychiatry is not available (Medical Group Management Association 2018).

The mean debt of graduating medical students in 2019, most of which is attributable to medical education, was $201,490. These figures do not include the accumulating interest that occurs during residency (Agapoff et al. 2018). Forty-four percent of graduating medical students currently opt to enter loan-forgiveness or repayment programs (Association of American Medical Colleges 2019). The desire to enter such programs as soon as possible to defray interest is another potential deterrent to fellowship training.

## Institutional Challenges

Institutions differ regarding funding fellowship positions, administrative support staff, and program directors' protected time. Some GME offices are reluctant to financially support subspecialty training. Many fellowship programs cannot financially support interview perks such as restaurant meals, travel expenses, or memorabilia. In some programs, funding for fellowships may be tenuous and inconsistent.

## Cultural Considerations

Fellowship directors should be mindful of the recommendations and efforts supported by the Liaison Committee of Medical Education and the

ACGME regarding diversity and inclusion. One aspect of diversity directly impacting fellowships is that IMGs are less likely to match into psychiatry compared with 5 years ago (Accreditation Council for Graduate Medical Education 2019b). Fewer IMGs in the fellowship applicant pool may impact fellowship recruitment downstream because many of these positions have traditionally been filled by IMGs.

# FUTURE DIRECTIONS IN SUBSPECIALTY TRAINING

## Trends in Subspecialty Training

In recent years, interest in general psychiatry among U.S. medical students has increased sharply (Agapoff et al. 2018). It is unclear what effect increased interest will have on future fellowship fill rates. All psychiatric subspecialties must address the misperception that specialized fellowship training simply is not necessary and focus on the benefits of such training, including increased marketability and unique skill sets.

## "Balkanization" of Medicine

It may also be helpful to view the challenges facing the psychiatric subspecialties in light of the so-called Balkanization of medicine. By the end of the nineteenth century, collective knowledge of medicine had expanded to a degree that a single physician could not reasonably maintain adequate working knowledge, much less mastery, of the entire field (Weisz 2003). The prevailing logic was to cordon off diagnostically similar patients in a manner that afforded physicians exposure to as many "specialized" cases as possible. Since ophthalmology was approved as the first U.S. medical subspecialty in 1917, medicine has further divided into 24 member boards representing 40 specialties and 87 subspecialties.

At the specialty level, distinctions are easy to make. Orthopedic surgeons and immunologists are grossly dissimilar in their training, pathological focus, and treatments offered. At the subspecialty level, however, the distinctions are less clear. Although some subspecialties have carved out clear consultative territory (e.g., cardiology, infectious disease), a range of problems in these fields remain that generalists are comfortable managing. In many ways, the usefulness of the subspecialist is defined by the threshold at which the generalist no longer feels comfortable.

Applying this rationale to psychiatric subspecialties, child and adolescent psychiatry is perhaps positioned most favorably as being distinct from the field of general psychiatry. Accordingly, the American Academy of Child and Adolescent Psychiatry Regional Council voted overwhelmingly (100 to 3) in 2018 to explore a single-board, 4-year direct match into child and adolescent psychiatry residency (Harris 2018). No such initiatives exist with regard to the other four psychiatric subspecialties.

## Future of Psychiatric Fellowships

The ABPN convened a "Crucial Issues Forum" in 2014 to address potential problems facing subspecialties. The ABPN announced there would be no moratorium placed on developing new programs and noted that the option of beginning subspecialty training during the final year of general residency was viewed more favorably by psychiatrists as compared with neurologists.

Despite the prevailing 4-year approach to general psychiatry residency, many believe that current ACGME requirements for general psychiatry can be completed within 36 months (Balon 2017). The fourth year of psychiatry residency may provide meaningful developmental opportunities to residents through mentorship of junior trainees; longitudinal patient care, particularly in psychotherapy; and the pursuit of electives. Some have therefore suggested that residents should "fast-track" into all subspecialties as they may do with child and adolescent fellowships. Discussion of the advantages and disadvantages of shortening general residency training to offset the disincentive of longer training and increase recruitment to fellowships continues within the field.

## Potential Regulatory Measures

Regulatory changes could foster specialization within psychiatry. For example, some states require clinical psychologists to undergo specialized forensic training as a prerequisite to performing forensic evaluations. Similar "scope of practice" limitations may not neatly apply to the psychiatric subspecialties and could narrow access to care even further. A general psychiatrist addressing chemical dependency is not analogous to a family practitioner attempting interventional cardiology. With the exception of child and adolescent psychiatry, psychiatric fellowships remain in their relative infancy. The high demand for general and specialized psychiatrists makes the requirement for *additional* certification to practice within any branch of the field unlikely. As such, it is incumbent upon psychiatric subspecialists to continue strengthening the case that fellowship training provides meaningful, marketable skills beyond general residency.

# CONCLUSION

Although there are ongoing challenges, subspecialty training remains meaningful and rewarding. Sharing a passion for psychiatric subspecialty practice with their fellows, residents, and medical students is a highlight for many academic psychiatrists. Strong leadership and quality teaching will continue to shape each psychiatric subspecialty in the years ahead.

## — KEY POINTS —

- Despite recent increases in general psychiatry applications, psychiatric subspecialty applications have plateaued or in some cases declined.
- Fostering interest is imperative when recruiting for subspecialties; early subspecialty exposure in medical school and residency may be key to fostering early interest.
- Each psychiatric subspecialty faces unique challenges to maintaining wellness that need to be considered and taught to trainees.
- Subspecialty faculty should consider lecturing and becoming involved in the residency interview process, providing grand rounds, and participating in departmental committees.
- Psychiatric subspecialties must highlight the benefits of subspecialty training and counter misperceptions about the necessity of subspecialty training.

# REFERENCES

Accreditation Council for Graduate Medical Education: Common Program Requirements (One-Year Fellowship). Chicago, IL, Accreditation Council for Graduate Medical Education, 2019a. Available at: https://www.acgme.org/Portals/0/PFAssets/ProgramRequirements/CPROneYearFellowship2020.pdf. Accessed November 25, 2020.

Accreditation Council for Graduate Medical Education: Data Resource Book: Academic Year 2018–2019. Chicago, IL, Accreditation Council for Graduate Medical Education, 2019b. Available at: https://www.acgme.org/About-Us/Publications-and-Resources/Graduate-Medical-Education-Data-Resource-Book. Accessed October 19, 2019.

Accreditation Council for Graduate Medical Education: Number of accredited programs by academic year: 2019–2020. ACGME website, 2019c. Available at: https://apps.acgme.org/ads/Public/Reports/Report/3. Accessed October 19, 2019.

Agapoff JR, Olson DK: Challenges and perspectives to the fall in psychiatry fellowship applications. Acad Psychiatry 43:425–428, 2019

Agapoff JR, Tonai C, Eckert DM, et al: Challenges and perspectives to the rise in general psychiatry residency applications. Acad Psychiatry 42:674–675, 2018

American Academy of Child and Adolescent Psychiatry: What is child and adolescent psychiatry? AACAP website, 2019. Available at: https://www.aacap.org/aacap/Medical_Students_and_Residents/Medical_Students/What_is_Child_and_Adolescent_Psychiatry.aspx. Accessed September 22, 2019.

American Academy of Family Physicians: Mental Health Care Services by Family Physicians (Position Paper). AAFP website, 2018. Available at: https://www.aafp.org/about/policies/all/mental-services.html. Accessed September 28, 2019.

American Association of Directors of Psychiatric Residency Training: Subspecialty fellowship application information. 2019 Available at: https://www.aadprt.org/trainees/psychiatry-training#Subspecialty. Accessed November 25, 2020.

American Medical Association Council on Ethical and Judicial Affairs: Code of Medical Ethics of the American Medical Association (eBook). Chicago, IL, American Medical Association, 2017

Association of American Medical Colleges: Medical student education, debt, costs and loan repayment fact card (website). Association of American Medical Colleges, 2019. Available at: https://store.aamc.org/medical-student-education-debt-costs-and-loan-repayment-fact-card-2019-pdf.html. Accessed September 21, 2019.

Balon R: Subspecialty training: time for a change. Acad Psychiatry 41:558–560, 2017

Bentley PG, Kaplan SG, Mokonogho J: Relational mindfulness for psychiatry residents: a pilot course in empathy development and burnout. Acad Psychiatry 42:668–673, 2018

Brotheron SE, Etzel SI: Graduate medical education, 2017–2018. JAMA 320:1051–1070, 2018

Cherry DK, Schappert SM: QuickStats: percentage of mental health-related primary care office visits, by age group—national ambulatory medical care survey, United States, in 2010 National Ambulatory Medical Care Survey. MMWR Morb Mortal Wkly Rep 63(47):1118, 2014. Available at: https://www.cdc.gov/mmwr/preview/mmwrhtml/mm6347a6.htm. Accessed September 28, 2019.

Dean J: Increasing recruitment into child and adolescent psychiatry: a resident's perspective. Acad Psychiatry 41:243–245, 2017

Faulkner LR, Juul D, Andrade NN, et al: Recent trends in American Board of Psychiatry and Neurology psychiatric subspecialties. Acad Psychiatry 35:35–39, 2011

Harris JC: Meeting the workforce shortage: toward 4-year board certification in child and adolescent psychiatry. J Am Acad Child Adolesc Psychiatry 57:722–724, 2018

Juul D, Scheiber SC, Kramer TA: Subspecialty certification by the American Board of Psychiatry and Neurology. Acad Psychiatry 28:12–17, 2004

Kang M, Selzer R, Gibbs H, et al: Mindfulness-based intervention to reduce burnout and psychological distress, and improve wellbeing in psychiatry trainees: a pilot study. Australas Psychiatry 27:219–224, 2019

Kelly M, Hearn J, McBride A, et al: A guide for applying to forensic psychiatry fellowship. Acad Psychiatry 41(6):793–797, 2017

Kirwin P, Conroy M, Lyketsos C, et al: A call to restructure psychiatry general and subspecialty training. Acad Psychiatry 40:145–148, 2016

Medical Group Management Association: DataDive (website). Medical Group Management Association, 2018. Available at: https://data.mgma.com. Accessed October 21, 2019.

National Resident Matching Program: Results and Data: Specialties Matching Service, 2018 Appointment Year. Washington, DC, National Resident Matching Program, 2018. Available at: https://mk0nrmp3oyqui6wqfm.kinstacdn.com/wp-content/uploads/2018/02/Results-and-Data-SMS-2018.pdf. Accessed October 21, 2019.

National Resident Matching Program: Results and Data: Specialties Matching Service, 2019 Appointment Year. Washington, DC, National Resident Matching Program, 2019. Available at: http://www.nrmp.org/wp-content/uploads/2019/02/Results-and-Data-SMS-2019.pdf. Accessed September 15, 2019.

Tampi RR, Zdanys KF, Srinivasan S, et al: Advice on how to choose a geriatric psychiatry fellowship. Am J Geriatr Psychiatry 27:687–694, 2019

Waheed A, Sadhu J, Kerlek A, et al: The biopsychosocial model of program self-evaluation: an innovative and holistic approach to enhance child and adolescent psychiatry training and recruitment. Acad Psychiatry 43:542–546, 2019

Weisz G: The emergence of medical specialization in the nineteenth century. Bull Hist Med 77:536–575, 2003

## CHAPTER 15

# FACULTY AND CAREER DEVELOPMENT IN ACADEMIC PSYCHIATRY

Mary "Molly" Camp, M.D.
Adam Brenner, M.D.

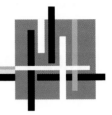

**In** this chapter, we review trends and best practices for faculty and career development in academic psychiatry. Broadly defined, *faculty development* refers to all activities that improve the knowledge, skills, and behaviors of health professionals related to their roles as educators, teachers, leaders, researchers, and scholars (Steinert et al. 2016). The Accreditation Council for Graduate Medical Education (ACGME) describes faculty development as a "structured program developed for the purpose of enhancing transference of knowledge, skill, and behavior from the educator to the learner" (Accreditation Council for Graduate Medical Education 2018). Although faculty and career development are highly interrelated, in this chapter we define *faculty development* as acquiring the knowledge and skills necessary to competently perform as a psychiatric clinical educator (e.g., teaching and scholarship) and *career development* as identifying and pursuing personal goals. The first half of the chapter reviews trends and best practices in faculty development programs. The second half is designed for individual faculty seeking career development information. We expect that the needs of program developers and individual participants are informed by one another and that resulting educational activities should be of mutual benefit.

# FACULTY DEVELOPMENT

The ACGME Common Program Requirements for residency mandate annual faculty development in educational skills, quality improvement and patient safety, fostering their own and residents' well-being, and patient care based on their own practice-based learning (Accreditation Council for Graduate Medical Education 2018). It is worth noting that this description goes beyond "teaching how to teach" into other domains of professional responsibility and practice. Table 15–1 provides some examples of potential faculty development topics under the broader categories outlined by the ACGME.

**Table 15–1.** Potential topics for faculty development

| |
|---|
| **Educational skill** |
| Theories of learning |
| Interactive and active teaching modalities |
| Principles and practices of assessment |
| How to give (and receive) feedback |
| **Quality improvement (QI) and patient safety** |
| Principles of QI |
| Implementation of a QI project |
| Dissemination of QI results |
| **Fostering well-being** |
| Fatigue management |
| Recognition and prevention of burnout |
| Reflection |
| **Patient care and practice learning** |
| Evaluation of practice habits and outcomes |
| Clinical and research updates for clinical care |
| **Other** |
| Curriculum development |
| Development and dissemination of scholarly projects |
| How to be an effective mentor and mentee |
| Leadership skill development |

In a comprehensive review of faculty development, McLean et al. (2008) provided a framework for considering which topics to teach and when. For instance, institutions might cover theories of learning, interactive teaching methods, principles of assessment, and delivering feedback for all teaching faculty. Based on individualized and site-specific needs, programs may include topics such as learning in the clinical environment, medical education research, writing for publication or grant proposals, leadership, or policy development, among others.

In recognition of the complex needs of academic psychiatrists, the American Association of Directors of Psychiatric Residency Training (AADPRT) created a Faculty Development Task Force in 2017. This task force began with a national survey of current practices, needs, and barriers for faculty development within psychiatric departments (De Golia et al. 2019). Among the general program directors responding, 91% reported having some sort of faculty development program in place in their department. Such programs were most often led by general program directors, chairs, or associate/vice chairs or directors of education. The most commonly reported activities were educational grand rounds, teaching workshops, and funding for external conferences. Sixty-eight percent of respondents identified the need for more protected time and additional training in teaching skills, and 83.9% expressed interest in a workshop on "How to Implement a Faculty Development Program." The second most-requested workshop was "How to Develop a Faculty Educational Scholarship Program." Program directors also indicated unmet needs for faculty development and the lack of a cohesive faculty development program in their institutions.

## Trends and Best Practices for Faculty Development

Faculty development occurs in a variety of formats, both formal and informal, group and individual, didactic and experiential (Steinert et al. 2016). Several principles emerge from the medical education literature describing the design of a high-quality, individualized program.

### *GENERAL AND TARGETED NEEDS ASSESSMENT*

As with any educational activity, faculty development activities must begin with a needs assessment. But whose needs should be considered?

In the six-steps approach outlined by Thomas et al. (2016), good curricular design begins with a general needs assessment that considers the broader "problem," the current approach, and an ideal approach. Considering faculty development, the "problem" may occur at a broader organizational level (e.g., ACGME requirements) or at a systems level (e.g., teaching faculty to balance educational and clinical responsibilities for residents). This type of needs assessment may ensure that programs are in good standing but does not ensure that the needs of the individual faculty will be appreciated and addressed.

A targeted needs assessment considers the unique needs of the individual learner or learning environment and should take into account factors such as the experience level of the learners and their involvement in education. For example, a new faculty member who teaches 1 day per week in a resident clinic will have very different needs than a professor who develops curriculum across the university. The individual career goals of the learner must also be considered. Unique factors of the educational setting will influence which topics should be covered and in what depth. Therefore, "broad strokes" approaches such as grand rounds on educational topics may address some faculty development needs but are limited in meeting the needs of individuals and will require supplementation with specialized learning activities, site-based teaching, or mentoring (McLean et al. 2008).

### *EVIDENCE-INFORMED TEACHING METHODS*

After assessing general and targeted needs, program developers should develop specific and measurable goals and objectives (Thomas et al. 2016). It is paramount to have a clear vision for what the program is trying to accomplish and to be able to evaluate whether objectives are being met. Faculty development programs are educational programs and require evaluation and revision to better meet objectives and to incorporate new ones based on the ever-changing needs of individuals and systems of care.

Faculty development programs should adhere to principles of adult learning and provide appropriate rigor to reach stated goals (Steinert et al. 2016). The literature describes myriad types of programs, from isolated workshops to yearlong fellowships (Leslie et al. 2013). Programs will likely need to incorporate multiple formats depending on specific objectives and learning environments. Developers should incorporate interactive learning modalities geared toward immediate actionable change in practice and provide methods for feedback as these changes are implemented. For instance, if faculty members struggle with writing informative narrative evaluations of trainees, a workshop can provide instruction and practice opportunities in this area, and the program then can compare faculty evaluations before and after the intervention to assess its effectiveness. Creating durable educational materials that can be used for future reference and promoting interdisciplinary collaborations may increase the impact of the educational effort (McLean et al. 2008).

### *LONGITUDINAL EXPOSURE*

Recent trends in faculty development advocate for longitudinal delivery of content. In their review, Steinert et al. (2016) found an increase in reports of longitudinal programs and a decrease in seminar series and workshops. As with other types of learning, professional development does not occur in a "one and done" fashion; ideally, learners should have opportunities to build on learning over time. Locally developed activities, scholars' programs or fellowships, or programming with national organizations may provide such opportunities. As an example, the Association for Academic Psychiatry offers a "Master Educator" track, a multiyear training in medical education, at their annual meeting.

### *EXPANDED MODEL OF FACULTY DEVELOPMENT*

Some recent literature advocates for an "expanded model" of faculty development that considers broader context and community beyond the individual learner. O'Sullivan and Irby (2011) described faculty development as a "social enterprise" involving two communities: 1) the community created among the learners in the program and 2) the broader workplace community.

The first community, which includes the learners themselves, may provide valuable insights and resources that an individual learner in isolation may not access. Participants may benefit from learning with colleagues who provide collaboration and feedback. Interdisciplinary collaborations model positive practices that trainees should be encouraged to emulate.

The "workplace community" is a broader network of environments in which learning takes place for faculty. Professional learning may occur in a classroom; more often, professional and practice-based learning occurs in the workplace (O'Sullivan and Irby 2011). As educators translate acquired knowledge into skills, the workplace allows for improvement and advancement of educational skills and must provide some support for teaching in the form of time, physical space, and connection with others. Faculty developers should consider ways to connect the classroom and the workplace. For instance, classroom learning may incorporate some reflection on workplace dynamics, and workplace learning may incorporate some on-site educational activities. In this way, learners may be better able to translate their new knowledge into their unique practice and teaching environments.

### *INSTITUTIONAL SUPPORT*

Effective faculty development requires investment of time and money. When institutions do not have structured faculty development programs, faculty may advocate for more opportunities. First, faculty may

**Table 15–2.** Resources for faculty and career development

| Resource | Offerings |
|---|---|
| Accreditation Council for Graduate Medical Education | Webinars, online trainings, and posting of national meetings (www.acgme.org) |
| Association of American Medical Colleges (AAMC) | Resources for professional development (www.aamc.org/professional-development) |
| MedEdPortal | Peer-reviewed open-access resource for curricula through the AAMC (www.mededportal.org) |
| American Association of Directors of Psychiatric Residency Training | Annual meeting, online Virtual Training Office, and email listserv for members (www.aadprt.org) |
| Association for Academic Psychiatry | Annual meeting, including Master Educator track (www.academicpsychiatry.org) |
| Association of Directors of Medical Student Education in Psychiatry | Annual meeting and online training modules (www.admsep.org) |

collectively advocate for needs and opportunities and provide feedback on existing faculty development. For institutional leaders, an empowered faculty can serve as a tremendous asset for broader institutional investment. Second, program developers and individual faculty should look outside of the institution. Table 15–2 provides examples of online and national resources that can reduce the local investment required. Third, programs can encourage and create avenues for mentorship among faculty locally or across institutions that may enhance or form a framework for a successful plan.

# BUILDING A CAREER IN PSYCHIATRY EDUCATION

In this section, we outline some elements of building a career in psychiatric education. Specific resources for some topics exist, and the *Handbook of Career Development in Academic Psychiatry and Behavioral Sciences*, edited by Roberts and Hilty (2017), is an invaluable general reference.

## Choice of a Job

The way to become a psychiatric educator is not as clear as the path to residency or board certification. One of the first questions is, what type of job should you take to best become an educator? Although obvious, you should take a job that includes teaching opportunities. Working on a team with daily supervisory responsibilities for medical students and residents will quickly give you a great deal of experience.

## Teaching Opportunities and Time Management

Most career paths in medical education are grounded in successful teaching, so developing a reputation as a strong teacher is critical. Natural aptitude is important, but dedication to learning the skills critical to adult learning is at least equally so. Make time to attend any training for teachers that is offered. Ask for both confirmatory and corrective feedback directly from your learners. Ask experienced teachers to observe your teaching. Openness to feedback is key in developing skills and finding your own voice.

Elective teaching opportunities will often be available, such as leading small groups or seminars or evaluating observed structured clinical examinations and clinical skills verifications. The needs of your clinical work and personal life will often compete with career needs. It is the responsibility of the department and the institution to make sure you have adequate time to teach, but you generally must demonstrate dedication to and a passion for teaching before a department will invest financially in supporting time specifically for education. Investing uncompensated time, especially early in a career, develops the reputation of being a committed, generous, and effective teacher. When you decline teaching opportunities, let the requester know if you would consider them in the future. Often, faculty defer opportunities when their children are young and make it clear that they wish to participate at another time. Leaders must appreciate the personal and family needs of their faculty and allow individual faculty to develop professionally on different timelines. Mentors may be an invaluable resource regarding balancing such individual choices.

Priority setting and time management are critical skills to develop early. Stephen Covey (2013), author of *The 7 Habits of Highly Effective People*, provided several rubrics: Write a personal mission statement to articulate career goals, and with each project "begin with the end in mind," meaning focus initially on these goals. Covey suggested dividing tasks into a four-box grid. On the left side, boxes are marked "Not urgent" and "Urgent," and across the top, boxes are marked "Important" and "Not Important." Urgent/Important tasks get immediate attention, and the others are reasonably deferred until time permits. The great difficulty for most people are these other categories. For example, tasks that fall into the Urgent/Not Important box may expand to fill all of one's available time. A look at anyone's email inbox can provide plenty of examples. Important/Not Urgent tasks include recognizing opportunities, planning, relationship building, and developing our own capacities—items such as "developing lecture skills" or "writing a paper about that education innovation." Career development is significantly enhanced by actively identifying Important/Not Urgent tasks and making concrete commitment to their pursuit.

## Mentoring

Mentoring is a professional relationship whose goal is the career development and fulfillment of the mentee. The available evidence indicates that mentoring in academic medicine leads to greater subjective sense of personal development and career satisfaction. Mentoring results in increased research productivity and improved faculty retention, and some preliminary evidence indicates that mentored faculty reach promotion milestones earlier. Mentors may create opportunities by including a mentee on their own projects or working on a mentee's proposal or project. Effective mentors help with networking within the department, locally, and nationally (Guerrero and Brenner 2016).

Departments should facilitate matching junior faculty with senior faculty mentors. Although mentoring is a deeply generative and satisfying experience, time and productivity pressures mean that incentives must exist. Mentoring should be explicitly credited for promotion.

Senior educators in other specialties can be valuable mentors. The challenges of building an education career are often similar across departments. Offices dedicated to fostering the development of women faculty or faculty from underrepresented groups may provide excellent potential mentors. You also may find mentors through meetings of national organizations, such as the Association of Directors of Medical Student Education in Psychiatry, Association for Academic Psychiatry, and AADPRT, some of which have formal mentoring matching programs.

## Moving Into Management

Confidence and experience may lead to ideas regarding how courses should be constructed and managed, and developing new curricula will showcase your capabilities. It is not always easy to think in terms of self-promotion and reputation management. A teacher's role focuses on the needs and, hopefully, promotion of the learners. In the long run, managing curricula will improve the experience for your learners.

## Compensation

In most academic medical settings, teaching and supervising are considered an intrinsic part of the job and therefore already compensated. Clinical productivity and documentation demands may make this less than fair. However, in most institutions, additional compensation is unusual without a significant education leadership or management role. Occasionally, education roles have an established compensation structure. Some departments and institutions have clear and consistently applied ways of financially supporting education time, such as compensation for a percentage of time or giving a bonus. If an educational leadership role is not compensated or is newly established, you must negotiate your compensation with the chair or the dean's office (Brenner et al. 2018).

Anxiety about negotiation is typically amplified by a lack of any explicit instruction during medical school or residency. Fortunately, you can teach yourself negotiation or learn it from a mentor. *Getting to Yes* is a timeless classic as a starting point (Fisher et al. 2011). Negotiation skills are a frequent topic of workshops at meetings of national education organizations. For example, suppose you are meeting with the chair to propose a new course that you will direct. You must focus on why this course is in the interest of the department—how it advances the educational mission and the current priorities of the chair. You must consider the current priorities of the department: Are they most concerned with recruiting more medical students into psychiatry, increasing residents' scholarship, or promoting community engagement/advocacy? Each of these will give you leverage in negotiation.

## Understanding and Preparing for Academic Promotion

Academic promotion, the process of moving to a higher academic rank, is often independent of workplace role or job title. The importance and difficulty of attaining promotion differ across institutions; departments prioritize and support promotion differently as well. It is in your interest to pursue promotion. It may raise your salary and will generally raise your reputation on campus, especially with other specialty physicians and departments.

Begin with a careful examination of the criteria and process for promotion. Ask senior department mentors about their experience with the promotion process. If you are asked to write the first draft of your promotion letter, obtain other examples. Begin to collect materials for promotion on your first day (or start now). Create folders, electronic and physical, to keep all evaluations and performance metrics. Notes from appreciative residents or students may provide quotations for your promotion letter. Keep an up-to-date curriculum vitae on your desktop and add elements to this document as they happen. Forward any positive feedback that you receive to those overseeing your education work; this could include the clerkship or program director, the vice chair for education, or the chair, who should be informed that you are successfully advancing the missions of the department and therefore on track for promotion.

Academic medical centers differ on whether they require scholarly activity for promotion of clinician educators. If it is not required, it is valued. Such activity includes writing peer-reviewed professional publications but may also include presenting at conferences, reviewing for journals, and writing for nonprofessional audiences. Determine the specific requirements and expectations at your institution.

## Developing Leadership Skills

The myth that particularly dynamic individuals simply have a "gift" for leadership is not true. Leaders have a set of skills that can be learned and developed. These skills include personnel management and leading change processes.

In overseeing education programs, you will interact differently with administrative personnel. Instead of being in a receptive mode—told when, where, and what to do—you will give such direction to others. This role is generally one for which most of us are unprepared. The quantity and quality of administrative support available are critical for your efficiency and effectiveness. You will have more time to teach if an administrative staff member performs some of your other tasks; this is much more cost effective.

Consultation from senior faculty, who can tell you about the work culture of the administrative personnel, may help you be a more effective supervisor. Engagement, autonomy, reward for initiative, and the like may be very different between professional worlds, even within the same department and institution. Because staff rarely support just one course, program, or faculty member, they may feel pulled in multiple conflicting directions when setting priorities. It is usually best to talk about conflicting priorities directly. Simply saying "I hope this can be done by the end of the week, but I know you support several faculty members, so please tell me if that is realistic," conveys respect and helps with workflow.

Change management is a constant in a career in education. New mandates from the institution or regulatory agencies, as well as creative and innovative ideas that will improve your classes, will bring people together to create change. The first task in managing change is to identify all the stakeholders in the current system: Who will experience an impact from this change? The next task is to reflect on the interests and motivations of all involved. Effective leadership aligns everyone's intentions to work toward a common goal. Discussions about the benefits of this change for organizations or individual stakeholders may help the group make some sacrifices for a greater mission.

# CONCLUSION

Faculty and career development offer many exciting opportunities for growth and advancement of both individuals and their broader workplace communities. Each requires considering the broader community and context as well as personal needs and the broader systems in which those needs occur. We hope that by providing a framework for considering these issues, this chapter serves as a resource and a jumping-off place for additional consideration of these important topics.

## — KEY POINTS —

- A high-quality faculty development program considers the general needs of the organization as well as the specific needs of learners in the context of their working environments.
- Programs should adhere to evidence-informed principles of curriculum development and adult learning, and the scope should extend to the broader workplace.
- Career development involves vigorous but selective pursuit of opportunities to develop as a teacher and to distinguish oneself as an educator.
- Mentorship is essential, as is learning key leadership skills such as negotiation, personnel management, and driving change.

# REFERENCES

Accreditation Council for Graduate Medical Education: ACGME Common Program Requirements (Residency). Chicago, IL, Accreditation Council on Graduate Medical Education, 2018. Available at: https://www.acgme.org/Portals/0/PFAssets/ProgramRequirements/CPRResidency2019.pdf. Accessed March 29, 2020.

Brenner AM, Beresin EV, Coverdale JH, et al: Time to teach: addressing the pressure on faculty time for education. Acad Psychiatry 42:5–10, 2018
Covey SR: The 7 Habits of Highly Effective People: Powerful Lessons for Personal Change. New York, Simon and Schuster, 2013
De Golia SG, Cagande CC, Ahn MS, et al: Faculty development for teaching faculty in psychiatry: where we are and what we need. Acad Psychiatry 43:184–190, 2019
Fisher R, Ury W, Patton B: Getting to Yes: Negotiating Agreement Without Giving In. New York, Penguin, 2011
Guerrero APS, Brenner AM: Mentorship: a return to basics. Acad Psychiatry 40:422–423, 2016
Leslie K, Baker L, Egan-Lee E, et al: Advancing faculty development in medical education: a systematic review. Acad Med 88(7):1038–1045, 2013
McLean M, Cillers F, Van Wyk JM: Faculty development: yesterday, today, and tomorrow. Med Teach 39:555–584, 2008
O'Sullivan PS, Irby DM: Reframing research on faculty development. Acad Med 86:421–429, 2011
Roberts LW, Hilty DM: Handbook of Career Development in Academic Psychiatry and Behavioral Sciences, 2nd Revised Edition. Washington, DC, American Psychiatric Publishing, 2017
Steinert Y, Mann K, Anderson B, et al: A systematic review of faculty development initiatives designed to enhance teaching effectiveness: a 10-year update: BEME Guide No 40. Med Teach 38(8):769–786, 2016
Thomas PA, Kern DE, Hughes MT, et al (eds): Curriculum Development for Medical Education: A Six-Step Approach, 3rd Edition. Baltimore, MD, Johns Hopkins University Press, 2016

# GLOSSARY OF ACRONYMS

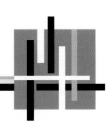

**AAAP**
American Academy of Addiction Psychiatry (www.aaap.org)

**AACAP**
American Academy of Child and Adolescent Psychiatry (www.aacap.org)

**AACDP**
American Association of Chairs of Departments of Psychiatry (www.aacdp.org)

**AADPRT**
American Association of Directors of Psychiatric Residency Training (www.aadprt.org)

**AAHC**
Association of Academic Health Centers (www.aahc.org)

**AAMC**
Association of American Medical Colleges (www.aamc.org)

**AAN**
American Academy of Neurology (www.aan.com)

**AAP**
Association of Academic Psychiatry (www.academicpsychiatry.org)

**AAPL**
American Academy of Psychiatry and the Law (www.aapl.org)

**ABIM**
American Board of Internal Medicine (www.abim.org)

**ABMS**
American Board of Medical Specialists (www.abms.org)

**ABPN**
American Board of Psychiatry and Neurology (www.abpn.com)

**ACGME**
Accreditation Council for Graduate Medical Education (www.acgme.org)

**ACP**
American College of Psychiatrists (www.acpsych.org)

**ADMSEP**
Association of Directors of Medical Student Education in Psychiatry (www.admsep.org)

**AHA**
American Hospital Association (www.aha.org)

**AHRQ**
Agency for Healthcare Research and Quality (www.ahrq.gov)

**AMA**
American Medical Association (www.ama-assn.org)

**APA**
American Psychiatric Association (www.psych.org)

**APM**
Academy of Psychosomatic Medicine (www.apm.org)

**APsaA**
American Psychoanalytic Association (www.apsa.org)

**AWP**
Association of Women Psychiatrists (www.associationofwomenpsychiatrists.com)

**CAS**
Council of Academic Societies (www.aamc.org/about/cas)

**CLER**
Clinical Learning Environment Review (www.acgme.org/What-We-Do/Initiatives/Clinical-Learning-Environment-Review-CLER)

**CMHS**
Center for Mental Health Services (www.mentalhealth.org)

**CMS**
Center for Medicare and Medicaid Services (http://cms.hhs.gov)

**CMSS**
Council of Medical Specialty Societies (www.cmss.org)

**CSV**
clinical skills verification

**DHHS**
U.S. Department of Health and Human Services (www.hhs.gov)

**DIO**
designated institutional official

**DoD**
U.S. Department of Defense (https://dod.defense.gov)

**EAM**
experiences, attributes, and metrics

**EAP**
Employee Assistance Program

**ECFMG**
Educational Commission on Foreign Medical Graduates (www.ecfmg.org)

**EMR**
electronic medical record

**ERAS**
Electronic Residency Application Service. AAMC software through which applicants build their applications and apply to programs. (www.aamc.org/services/eras-for-institutions/program-staff)

**FREIDA**
Fellowship and Residency Electronic Interactive Database (https://freida.ama-assn.org/Freida/#/)

**FSMB**
Federation of State Medical Boards (www.fsmb.org)

**GAP**
Group for the Advancement of Psychiatry (https://ourgap.org)

**GME**
graduate medical education

**HIPAA**
Health Insurance Portability and Accountability Act (www.hhs.gov/hipaa/index.html)

**IMG**
international medical graduate

**IRB**
institutional review board

**LCME**
Liaison Committee on Medical Education (www.lcme.org)

**MSPE**
Medical Student Performance Evaluation (www.aamc.org/professional-development/affinity-groups/gsa/medical-student-performance-evaluation)

**NBME**
National Board of Medical Examiners (www.nbme.org)

**NRMP**
National Residency Matching Program. "The Match" uses students' and certified programs' rank order lists to "match" programs and applicants. (www.nrmp.org)

**OSCE**
Objective Structured Clinical Examination

**PDWS**
Program Director Work Station. Part of ERAS that provides a portal for review of applications, communication with applicants, and scheduling of interviews.

**PGY**
postgraduate year

**PRITE**
Psychiatry Resident-In-Training Examination (www.acpsych.org/prite)

**RRC**
Residency Review Committee

**SOAP**
Supplemental Offer and Acceptance Program (www.nrmp.org/match-week-soap-applicants/)

**TOEFL**
Test of English as a Foreign Language (www.ets.org/toefl)

**UME**
undergraduate medical education

**USMLE**
United States Medical Licensing Examination (www.usmle.org)

**VA**
U.S. Department of Veterans Affairs

# Index

Page numbers printed in **boldface** type refer to tables and figures.